It's Your Life

End the confusion from inconsistent health advice

Professor Norman Ratcliffe

Swansea University

Wales, UK

Cranmore Publications

*A catalogue record for this book is available from
the British Library*

Illustrated by Hannah Michael

ISBN: 978-1-907962-11-0

Published by Cranmore Publications

Reading, England

www.cranmorepublications.co.uk

ACKNOWLEDGEMENTS

This book is dedicated to my parents whose undying faith in my academic capabilities allowed me to pursue a scientific career. My gratitude also goes to my sister, Teri King, whose success as an author and constant encouragement and advice were such sources of inspiration. Thanks too to my many friends for tolerating so many mealtime discussions on health and diet as well as the unsolicited advice given to them!

Finally, I wish to thank Dr. Duncan McLaren of Swansea Metropolitan University for his outstanding enthusiasm and imagination during creation of sections of this book as well as Doreen Montgomery of Rupert Crew Ltd for her patient and helpful comments of the manuscript.

"IT'S YOUR LIFE"

HOW TO USE THIS BOOK

- FED UP WITH CONTRADICTORY HEALTH/DIET ADVICE? NOT MUCH TIME AND JUST WANT THE BASIC FACTS?

- THEN DON'T READ THIS BOOK COVER TO COVER.

- JUST IDENTIFY CHAPTERS OF INTEREST FROM THE CONTENTS PAGES.

- READ THE SUMMARIES AT THE END OF MANY CHAPTERS AND/OR THE SECTION MOST APPROPRIATE TO YOUR AGE AND LIFESTYLE.

- WANT MORE DETAILS THEN READ THE REST OF THE CHAPTER AS REQUIRED.

- REMEMBER, YOUR PARTICULAR CONCERNS CAN BE ADDRESSED HERE.

- FOR EXAMPLE, YOU CAN FIND OUT AT A GLANCE:

i.   Which foods contain excess calories, saturated fats, sugar and salt (Chapter 2)

ii.   Which organic foods are most important to buy (Chapter 4)

iii. How to avoid pesticide-contaminated food (Chapter 4)

iv.   How to avoid the most dangerous food additives (Chapter 5)

v.   Your "Body Burden" of chemicals and their avoidance/elimination (Chapter 6)

vi.   Which vitamins are essential for your age group (Chapter 8)

vii. Which types of exercises are best for your age (Chapter 11)

"IT'S YOUR LIFE"
THE AUTHOR

- **Professor Norman Ratcliffe** is a founder member of a team that recently discovered a new antibiotic potentially capable of curing MRSA and *Clostridium difficile*. This work was presented to Prince Phillip at St. James's Palace, London and was the subject of major media attention in the UK on ITV News and in many leading newspapers, including the Wall Street Journal, around the World. He is a Fellow of the Royal Society of Medicine and has previously run a "Health Alert" blood-testing company. He has published over 200 books and research papers on immunology, cancer invasion, influenza, tropical diseases and MRSA. He played squash for Wales, ran the London Marathon at the age of 50 and works-out regularly in the gym.

- **Professor Ratcliffe** retired recently after 25 years as a University Research Professor. He decided to finally complete "It's Your Life" after 5 years work in order to help the many people who are confused about health and fitness issues and who have constantly been asking his advice.

"IT'S YOUR LIFE"
THE AIMS

- **The main aim of "IT'S YOUR LIFE" is to end the confusion** resulting from the huge outpouring of conflicting health advice appearing in the media almost daily. For example: Should we drink tap or bottled water? Is it necessary to buy solely organic foods? Are we being poisoned by pesticides and food additives? Are vitamin supplements really necessary and which ones should we take? Do we have to exercise 5 times per week? All advice offered is based on the analysis of existing scientific evidence and does not result from any alliance to a Government Organisation, an Alternative Health or Lifestyle Charity, or a Pharmaceutical Company. This book does not profess to tell you how to live to be a 100 years old but it does show you, SIMPLY, how to maintain health, fitness, strength, energy and a feeling of well-being throughout your life and into your later years.

- **"IT'S YOUR LIFE" also aims to change our present concepts and prejudices** that often compartmentalise people into certain categories at specific ages. Why is it that even well-meaning advertisements often portray 40+ people as unattractive and generally 50+ people as old, toothless, inactive and one step from the nursing home? The problem is that people are exposed to so much of this stereotyping that they subconsciously believe the hype and begin to live their lives accordingly.

WHAT IS SAFE AND WHO DO YOU BELIEVE?

High Levels?	
Medium Levels?	
Low Levels?	Very Low Levels?

OF FATS, FIBRE, PESTICIDES, ADDITIVES, VITAMINS, EXERCISE ETC
FIND OUT HERE!

"IT'S YOUR LIFE" IS A UNIQUE CONTRIBUTION SINCE:

- **It is for people of all different ages,** aiming to optimise health and fitness and maximise an active and independent lifestyle throughout life. It is not a part of the recent deluge of health and diet books or videos produced by B-class "celebrities" but has been written by a biomedical scientist of international repute.

- You will not find in most books **high impact illustrations** emphasising important points in the text. For example, the cover illustrates the present-day frustration and confusion of the average consumer exposed to contradictory health and dietary advice.

- You will not find in most books on diet and exercise clear summaries of **basic facts for adopting a new health plan.** Thus, for the many people with busy lives who may hate reading health books Chapter 1 ("Food, The Basic Diet"), Chapter 9 ("Exercise, Basic Introduction") and other Chapters are designed for rapid reference, often to specific age-groups of people.

- You will also not find in most other books descriptions of how many aspects of **diet and exercise change at different times of life** (Chapter 1) as well as reasons for weight gain as we age and advice as how to avoid this (Chapter 2, "Help! What Am I Eating?").

- You will also not find in most other books **extensive tables for rapid identification of foods containing high levels of calories, saturated fats, salt and sugar** (Chapter 2). Thus, information on over 300 different food groups can be extracted at a glance without the necessity of reading minute and confusing Supermarket Food Labels.

- You will also not find in most books **not only clearly tabulated facts** about **"The Good, The Bad And The Ugly Fats",** and **"Fibre"** but also appraisals of the Atkins and GI **"Fad Diets"** (Chapter 3).

- You will also not find in other books **details of the rates of pesticide contamination of fruit, vegetables and other types of food** using easily interpreted tables (Chapter 4). A summary table is also included, for attaching to the refrigerator door or notice board, to identify **the least chemically polluted foods.**

- You will also not find in other books **a list of organic foods that are the most important to buy** (Chapter 4) and an explanation why, in these financially challenged times, it is **unnecessary** to eat just organic foods.

- You will also not find in many other books **details of the potential impact on food safety of Food Additives, Preservatives and Colourants** (Chapter 5) together with consideration of the **total chemical loading** of the body from all sources (Chapter 6, "The Cocktail Effect"). Possible interactions of chemicals accumulated from pesticides and additives in food, and from cosmetics and household sources, are also discussed, and advice is given on **reducing the uptake of chemicals from the environment**.

- You will also not find in other books an understanding of the **"Vitamin Dilemma"** as **"To Take Or Not To Take, That Is The Question"** (Chapters 7 and 8) facing most people following conflicting advice in the media. Clear scientific analysis of the latest research shows that people require different supplements at different stages in their lives. **Supplement recommendations are made for each stage from pregnancy to old age.**

- You will also not find in most other books **an understanding of the "To Gym Or Not To Gym-That Is The Question" dilemma faced by many people beginning to exercise for the first time** (Chapter 9). It introduces the basics and benefits of regular exercise, describes how to begin training in the gym, and provides an outline exercise programme (Chapter 10).

- You will also not find in most other books **details of "Alternative Types Of Exercise For Gym–Haters"** (Chapter 11), with different sports and activities described together with the calories used and **a table of the time taken with different sports to burn off highly calorific snacks.** Uniquely, the effects of each type of exercise are presented in terms of joint damage and cardiovascular function, and **advice on exercising at different ages** is also included.

- In summary, **"IT'S YOUR LIFE",** presents the best advice available for optimising health and fitness in a manner designed to enlighten and engage the non-expert reader.

"IT'S YOUR LIFE"

Contents

INTRODUCTION

A SIMPLE HEALTH PLAN

MIDDLE–AGE SPREAD, just look around it's everywhere. Can we avoid the weight-gain, diseases, degeneration and general malaise that often seem to accompany the aging process? Have you noticed, in recent years, how more and more young people appear middle-aged? Why are some diseases such as cancer of the colon and diabetes of such prominence now? Can we avoid these changes and diseases? This book does not profess to tell you how to live to be a 100 years old but it does show you, **SIMPLY,** how to maintain health and fitness and a feeling of well-being into your later years.

Figure 1.   Showing slim (left) and overweight (right) females for comparison. The tape measure never lies!

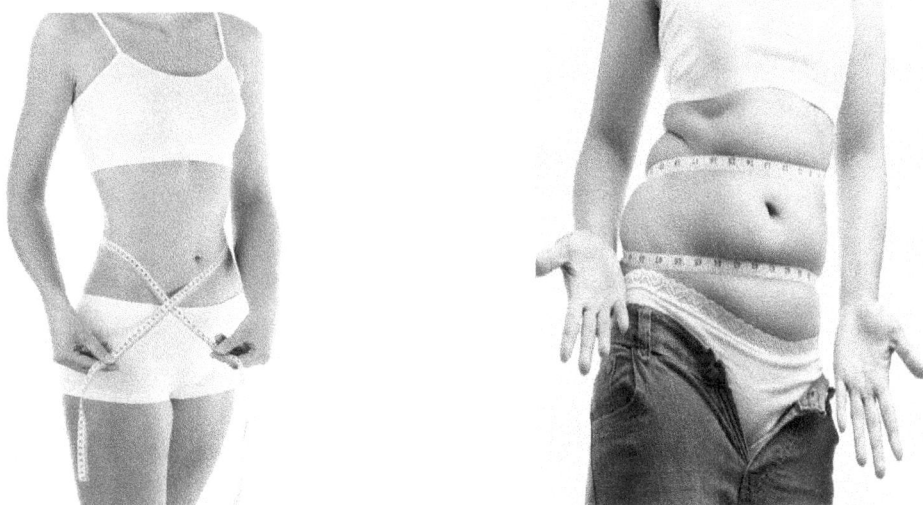

Figure 2. Showing slim (left) and over weight (right), middle-aged men for comparison

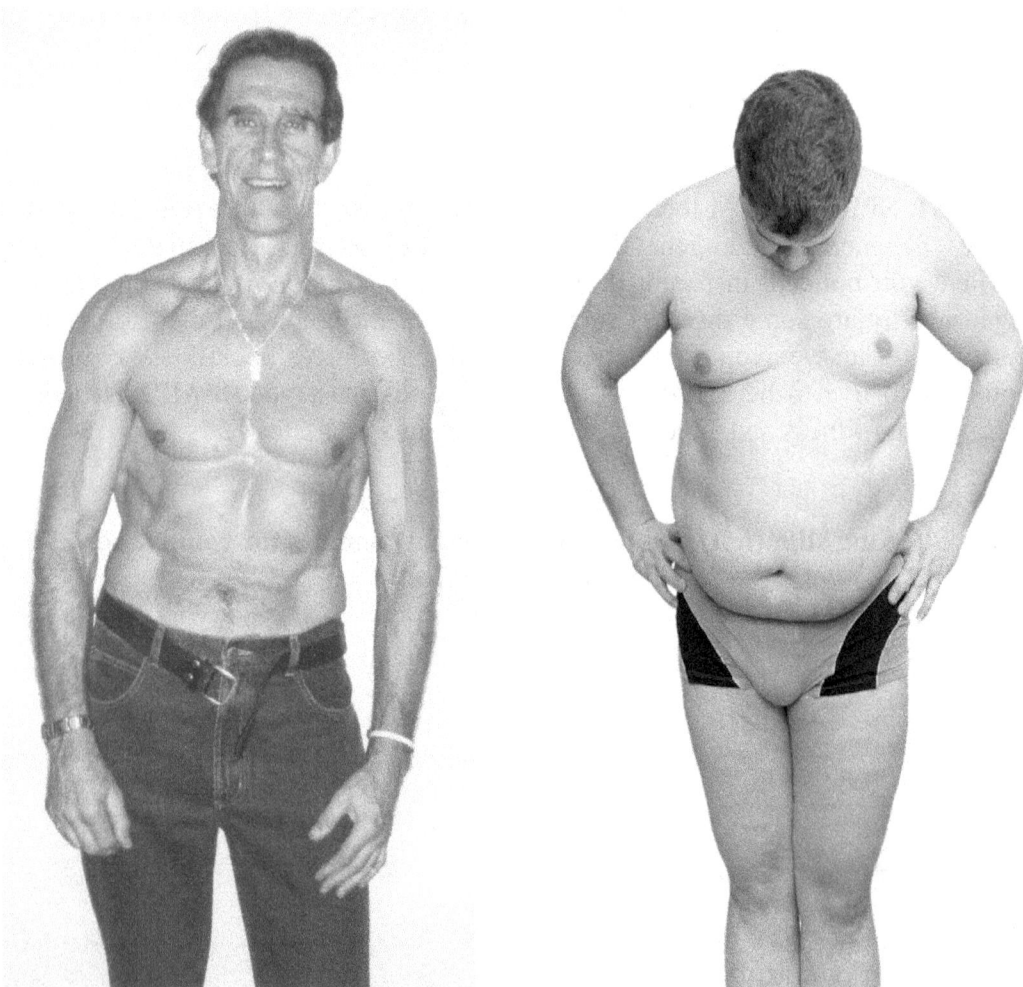

The author aged 65 yr

FED UP WITH THE CONSTANT BARRAGE OF HEALTH ADVICE AND DO'S AND DON'TS? The basics of a simple lifestyle are outlined on the next page. There is no need for you to read the entire book, you can simply try and follow the suggestions made in the 'Basic Health Plan'. If, however, you want to know more about the various components then the rest of the book will explain the details and will also introduce new health topics.

THE AGING PROCESS

Who knows why we age? Scientists have many theories including:

- Accumulation of damage to tissues by components of the oxygen that we breathe. Yes, oxygen can be poisonous to cells!

- Loss in ability of cells to multiply and self-repair due to changes in the aging chromosomes.

THE BASIC HEALTH PLAN

You have heard it all before from the media:

• Eat less junk-food and include 5 portions of fruit and vegetables in your diet each day
• Avoid too much animal fat and red meat - eat more fish and chicken
• Take regular exercise
• Give up smoking
• Avoid excess alcohol
• Examine your breasts, testicles and moles regularly for lumps and changes
• Get married

EASY TO SAY but how do you successfully change your lifestyle and end up with this desirable health plan? The following chapters will guide you **BUT REMEMBER :**

- If you hate reading health books then just concentrate on Chapters 1 ("Food, the basic diet") and 9 ("Exercise – basic introduction") as these are designed as an introduction to a new health plan.

- Chapters 2 and 3 ("More about food" and "More facts about food, fat, fibre and fad diets") enlarge on Chapter 1 and tell you details about calories and important food components as well as changing your diet with age.

- Chapters 10 and 11 describe how to begin an exercise programme.

CHAPTER 1

FOOD

The Basic Diet (not dieting)

THERE IS NO NEED TO PILE ON THE POUNDS PAST 40 YEARS OLD

- It's getting more and more difficult to walk up those stairs, carry the shopping bags any distance, kick the ball around or make love. It's time to **take control**.

- You have abused your body with greasy breakfasts, hamburgers, chips, crisps, pasties, cakes, fizzy drinks and ready meals so that the pounds are piling on and you don't bother much with vegetables and fruit so **what can you do**?

- The fact that you are reading this book is a good start and shows that you are concerned. The best start you can make is simply to understand that **you are eating too many calories** and as you get older the extra calories will turn into ugly fatty deposits and block your heart and blood vessels. **REMEMBER, YOU ARE WHAT YOU EAT.**

First, what about breakfast? Those fry-ups are delicious aren't they? Can you slowly reduce the number that you have each week? Maybe down to just one on Saturday morning. If this is difficult then try having a few more beans or tomatoes instead of all that bacon, those two eggs, fried bread, chips and fat-filled mushrooms. **USE THE TOMATO KETCHUP** (do not worry about snooty waiters). Ketchup is particularly good for men.

There is evidence that the red pigment, lycopene, an antioxidant found in tomatoes, and to a lesser extent in apricots, pink grapefruits, papayas and guavas, can protect against cancer of the prostate in men. A number of so-called "epidemiological studies" which looked at dietary intake of lycopene from tomatoes and tomato products and incidence rates of prostate cancer, found a reduced risk of cancer. One such study involved nearly 48,000 men over 12 years and reported that 2+ servings of tomato or tomato products per week significantly reduced prostate cancers rates (see reference 1).

Needless to say, there are other scientific studies that disagree about the protective properties of lycopene. The US Food and Drug Administration reviewed all these studies and concluded that there is "limited evidence to support an association between tomato consumption and reduced risks of prostate, ovarian, gastric, and pancreatic cancers" (see reference 2).

TOMATO SAUCE HAS PARTICULARLY HIGH LEVELS OF LYCOPENE which is highly concentrated during heating of the tomatoes to release this red pigment from the tissues. The oil base of the sauce assists lycopene absorption in the gut. Other food products containing high levels of lycopene include tomato juice, tomato paste, condensed tomato soup, pizza sauce, spaghetti and baked bean sauce and some barbecue sauces. Raw tomatoes are best cooked to release the lycopene.

Figure 1. Who says that a dog is man's best friend? Tomatoes contain high levels of the red pigment, lycopene, which can significantly reduce rates of prostate cancer in men

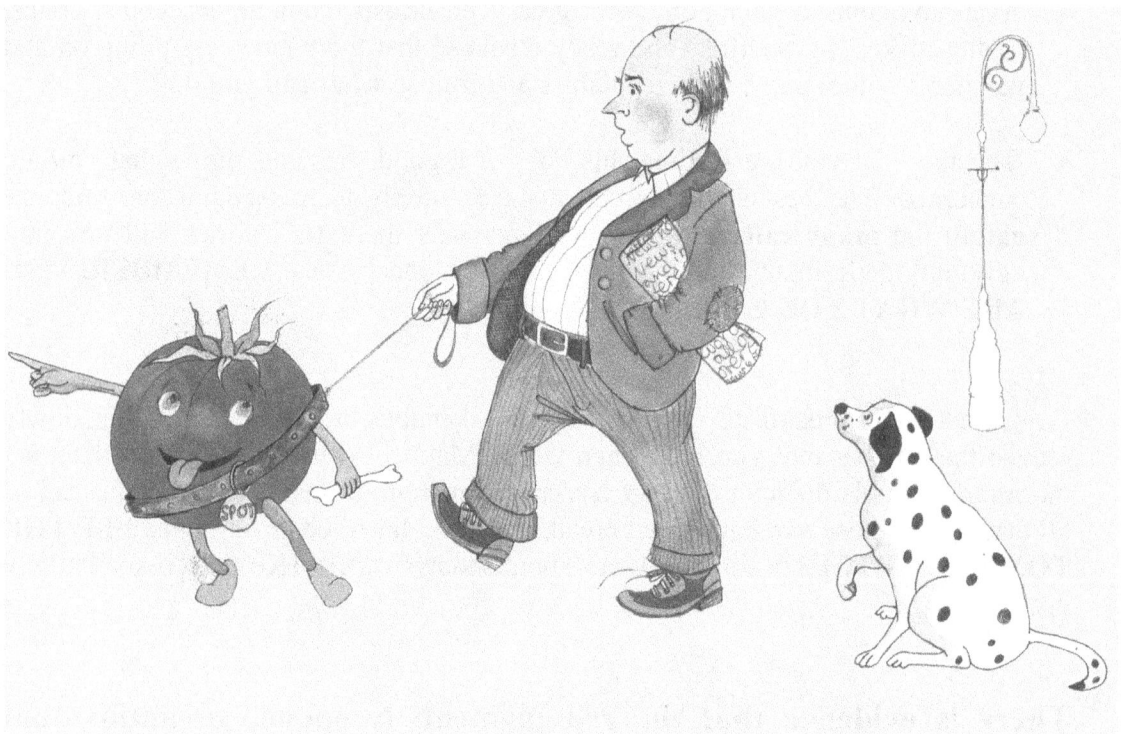

NEVER MISS BREAKFAST COMPLETELY as it is, as the name implies, the breaking of the overnight fasting and your blood sugar levels will be low. Your sugar levels will continue to fall and, unless you eat something, you will be tempted to snack mid-morning. What can you eat **instead of fried breakfasts or white toast with thick layers of butter or margarine or no breakfast at all?** Some cereal

(Weetabix, Shredded Wheat or unsweetened Muesli are much better than Sugar Puffs, Cornflakes, Rice Crispies or Coco Pops) with skimmed milk is good, maybe with a little toast (wholemeal is best) and marmalade/Marmite. Try the toast just with marmalade/jam/Marmite and you will soon forget about the butter/margarine. Significantly, Marks and Spencer are removing products made with **trans fats (=hydrogenated vegetable fats, causing heart problems, see Chapter 3 for details), including some MARGARINES, from the shelves.** Try and avoid whole milk in latte or cappuccino. When ordering a coffee in a restaurant, it is worthwhile asking what sort of milk is being used and requesting skimmed or semi-skimmed if possible.

If you are really determined to start anew then **OATMEAL PORRIDGE (** which has low fat and salt, and reduces cholesterol and stress) with skimmed milk and a little honey is great, not only for the heart but also will suppress the desire to snack later in the day.

The importance of breakfast for children cannot be over-emphasised. A recent survey of 213 children between the ages of 4 and 11 commissioned by Kellogg's entitled "The Effects of Cereal on Children" (detailed at **www.kelloggs.co.uk/mediacentre**) showed that children who eat cereal for breakfast are mentally more alert for school than children who skip breakfast. The benefits of eating breakfast cereal included:

Benefits of children eating breakfast cereal before school

- 9 percent more alert
- 11 percent less emotionally distressed
- 13 percent less tired
- 17 percent less anxious
- 10 percent less likely to suffer memory and attention span problems
- 33 percent less likely to suffer from stomach complaints

Eating breakfast results in higher concentration and energy levels, as well as improving behaviour and well-being in children.

Figure 2. Shows that eating breakfast results in higher concentration and better school work in children as well as increased energy levels and improved behaviour and well-being

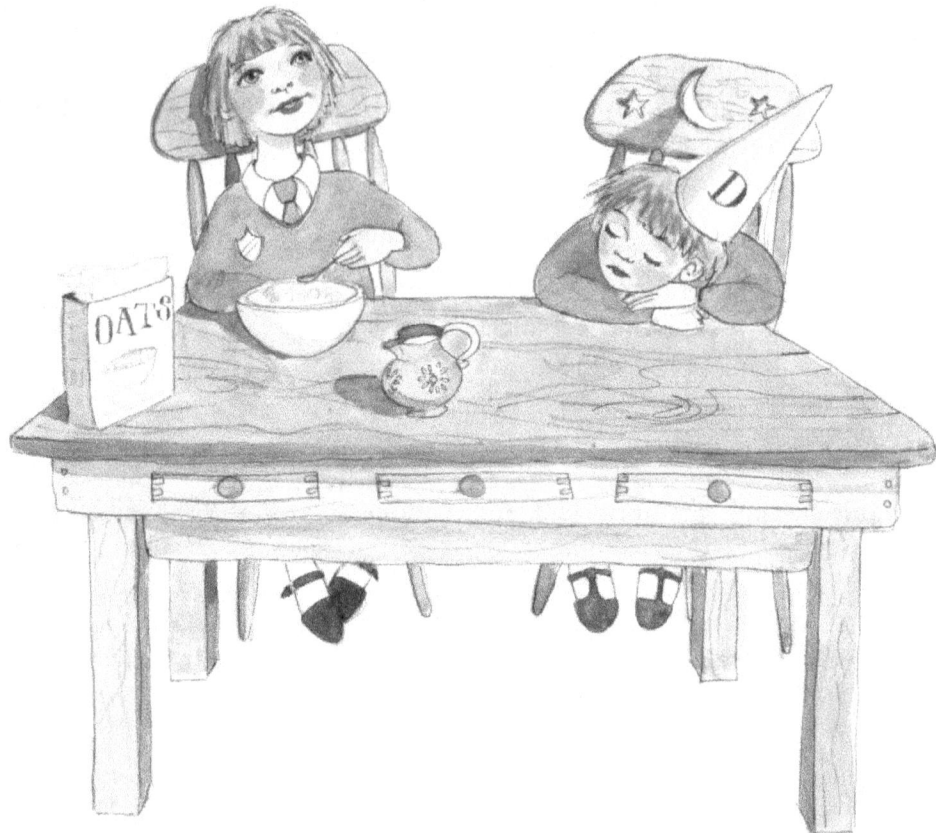

No, don't go on a **NEW FAD OR TRENDY DIET** that you read about in the newspaper or your favorite celebrity is promoting for money. First, just try replacing the fizzy drink with water or non-fizzy fruit juice (but not too many as juices contain calories too) and introduce an apple, orange, banana or a few grapes (any fruit!) into your diet each day. Once you succeed then look at the hamburger, cheeseburger, chips, meat pie, instant frozen meal or white roll etc that you normally eat and **consult the calorie chart (see Chapter 2, Table 1).** Do you really want all that processed high fat and salt-containing stodge or could you replace it with a few potatoes or rice (brown preferred) and a piece of cooked chicken or fish? Sounds boring but can be delicious with some pasta sauce on the chicken/fish cooked (not burnt) in a pan/oven with olive oil.

AVOID EATING RED MEAT EVERY DAY as it has been estimated that people who eat red meat twice instead of once per week have double the chance of developing bowel cancer. Recently, it has been shown that men who ate high amounts of red meat per week (about 6 oz or more =160 grams red meat per day) were 22% more likely to die from cancer and 27% more likely to die from heart disease than those who ate low amounts of red meat (about 1 oz = 25 grams) per day. In women, the equivalent figures for those who eat high amounts of red meat were 20% more likely to die of cancer and 50% more likely to die of heart disease, compared with women who consumed the lowest levels. Processed meats such as hotdogs, sausages and pepperoni were even worse than red meat (see reference 3).

By all means have a good steak or roast beef once a week. Red meat includes beef, lamb, bacon, gammon and pork, while white meats are chicken, turkey and fish. White meat should be eaten most days although the occasional omelette is fine.

FANTASTIC, YOU ARE WELL ON THE WAY.

Next try and include a few peas, beans, carrots (fresh cooked are delicious) or any vegetable you can stand with your meal. Yes, cooking is a chore so salad is fine or **buy a steamer** in which you can cook all the vegetables individually in the separate pans (retaining their vitamins) all at one time with minimal washing up (See Chapter 7, pages 148-9, for hints on the best methods of cooking to retain vitamins).

Again, but **especially men**, always use the ketchup freely (see pages 19-20 for reasons).

Whatever you do, try and watch the **amount of salt** that you are eating (see reference 4).

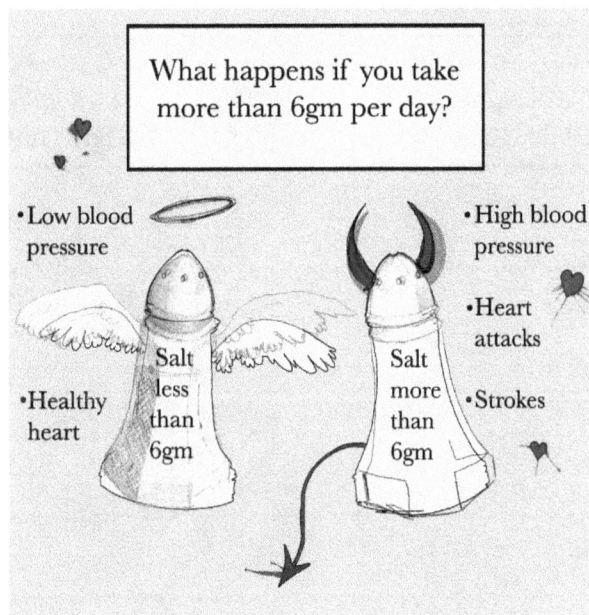

Figure 3. Shows that excess salt raises blood pressure and causes strokes and heart disease

The recommended daily amount is about 6 grams which is just more than one level teaspoon. Most salt is eaten in processed meals, crisps, bread, sauces and soup (see Chapter 2, Table 1, for salt contents of many foods). Read the labels on foods and remember the **"sodium" levels** shown have to be **multiplied by 2.5** in order to arrive at the true salt content. You will soon realize that a single instant meal often contains as much or even more than your 6 gram daily allowance! Thus, the limit on sodium intake is about 2.5 grams per day.

What about desserts? Have you tried **fresh fruit salad** (either bought from the supermarket or made by you) with some low fat yoghurt? You cannot stand yoghurt!? Ok, try the fruit salad alone or with a little custard or rice pudding (not made with full fat milk!). There is no fruit salad available? Ok, skip the rolly polly and chocolate puddings and buy some dried fruit and nuts instead.

Gradually, modify your diet, as above, until you will be surprised to find that you are eating at least the **"five portions of fruit or vegetables every day"** recommended by all doctors and nutritionists. These fruits and vegetables will contain most of the vitamins and minerals needed and all of the fibre required for a healthy gut (see Chapter 3 for more details on fibre).

Figure 4. Shows the benefits of eating at least 5 portions of fruit and vegetables per day

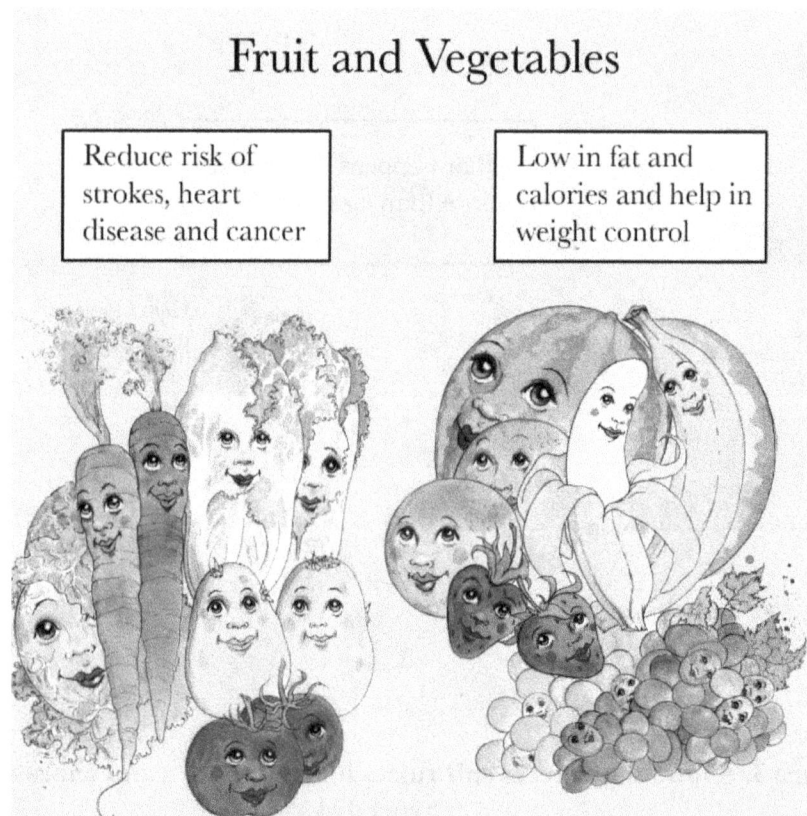

Fruit and Vegetables

Reduce risk of strokes, heart disease and cancer

Low in fat and calories and help in weight control

We are constantly told to eat 5 portions of fruit or vegetables per day for a number of reasons since they:

- Contain high levels of vitamins, minerals, fibre and antioxidants (see Chapters 3 and 7, for details)

- Are low in fat and calories and therefore help weight control

- May reduce the risk of strokes, heart disease and cancer

- Look attractive and stimulate the desire to eat healthily

LESS THAN 50% OF PEOPLE are aware of the need to eat 5 portions of fruit and vegetables every day. This is despite the constant reminder to do so by the media and health advisors.

EVEN FEWER PEOPLE know what makes up a portion of fruit or vegetable

SO WHAT IS A PORTION? It is no good being told to eat "5 portions" unless we know exactly what makes up a portion. According to the Food Standards Agency (**www.eatwell.gov.uk/healthydiet** and **www.5aday.nhs.uk/whatcounts**):

A PORTION OF FRUIT OR VEGETABLES = 80 g or just less than 3 ounces

However, we cannot weigh (especially in restaurants) all the fruit and vegetables that we eat so try remembering that **a portion** (fresh, tinned or frozen) is:

- 1 small glass (150ml or about 1/3 pint) of fruit or vegetable juice or smoothie* but fruit juice only counts as one portion no matter how many glasses you drink

- 2 smaller fruits such as plums, tangerines, kiwi fruits, or 3 apricots

- 1 medium fruit such as apple, pear, orange, nectarine or banana

- for larger fruits – ½ a grapefruit or avocado or 1 slice of melon or pineapple or 2 slices of mango (all about 2-inches thick)

- a handful of grapes, berries or dried fruit

- 3 heaped tablespoons of vegetables, chopped fruit or pulses (beans, peas, and lentils). Again, pulses only count as one portion no matter how much you eat

- A small dessert bowl of salad

* Smoothies are very fashionable and can be beneficial but **take care to check their ingredients** since they can have high sugar, fat and calorie contents. Also, most of the fibre has been removed and sometimes they are mixed with whole fat milk or yoghurt and not made with fresh fruit but fruit concentrate containing fewer vitamins and minerals. The famous American Peanut Butter Moo'd, marketed by Jumba Juice, contains chocolate and peanut butter and every 890ml packet has 1170 calories and 169 grams of sugars!

Potatoes are starchy foods and do not count towards your 5 portions per day.

If possible, drink a glass of red wine with dinner as it is good for the heart and circulation too.

DRINK PLENTY OF WATER throughout the day as it will help to detoxify the body, prevent dehydration, constipation and fatigue. Who counts how much they drink? However, about 6-8 average glasses of fluid per day is recommended and water, milk, teas, coffee, soup and fruit juices all count. Normal teas and coffees do tend to dehydrate the body and if your urine becomes dark yellow then drink some more water. The above 6-8 glasses of fluid per day apply whether you eat at home or in the canteen in work but do not count any alcohol.

THE TAP WATER VERSUS BOTTLED WATER DEBATE
See pages 33-36 of this chapter

Yes, the above looks like a diet but it is just sensible eating. The important thing is **NOT TO CHANGE EVERYTHING AT ONCE** but just pick those things that are easiest for you and introduce them slowly so that they become part of your normal daily routine. Following the advice above you should end up with a so-called **"Balanced Diet"**.

A balanced diet would include the following food groups:

1. **Bread, cereals, pasta, rice and potatoes** which are high in carbohydrate and called "starchy" foods. Carbohydrate should make up 50-60% of calories in diet.

2. **Fruit and vegetables** since these contain healthy carbohydrate, protein (pulses), fibre and vitamins.

3. **Meat** as a source of protein to include red meat, poultry, fish, eggs, and meat substitutes such as nuts and pulses (peas, beans and lentils). Avoid too much red meat (beef, pork, ham, lamb) and eat no more than 1-2 times per week. Protein to make up 15-25 % of calories in diet.

4. **Milk and dairy products** to include milk, cheese and yoghurt (all low-fat or skimmed) provide some protein, calcium and B vitamins and fats. Fats to make up 10-15% of calories in diet.

5. **Soft drinks and foods** such as sweets, jam, cakes, biscuits, puddings, crisps, ice cream and sauces all contain high added sugar and/or saturated fats and **should be limited and reduced if possible.**

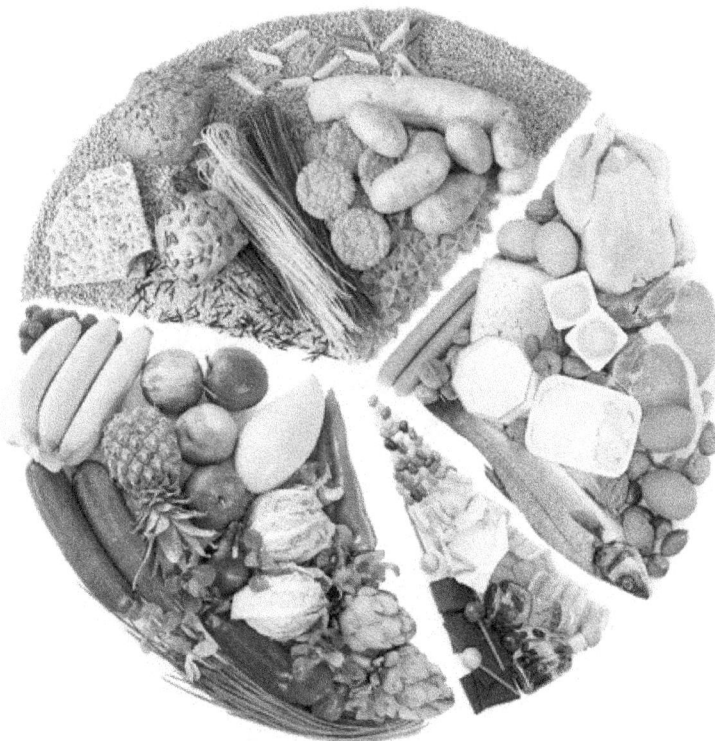

Figure 5. Shows the main groups of foods described above. The size of each slice represents the proportion of the diet that should contain that food group. Hence the smallest slice contains sweets, biscuits, cakes etc. Note that meat and dairy products have been combined into one slice

- A "balanced diet" would include a combination of foods from all of the main food groups (above) at each meal.

- Avoid foods high in saturated fat and trans fats as well as those with high levels of added sugar and salt (see Chapters 2 and 3).

- Beware added salt with a limit of 6 grams per day (= about one teaspoon full) or no more than 2.5 grams of sodium. This is confusing since sodium and not salt is often shown on food labels instead of salt (why do supermarkets do this?).

- There is no need to go on a special diet. Just gradually introduce healthy options into your diet to replace high fat, salt and sugar containing foods.

Figure 6. Shows junk food on the right-hand scale gradually being replaced by healthy fruit and vegetables on the left-hand scale to eventually arrive at a balanced diet

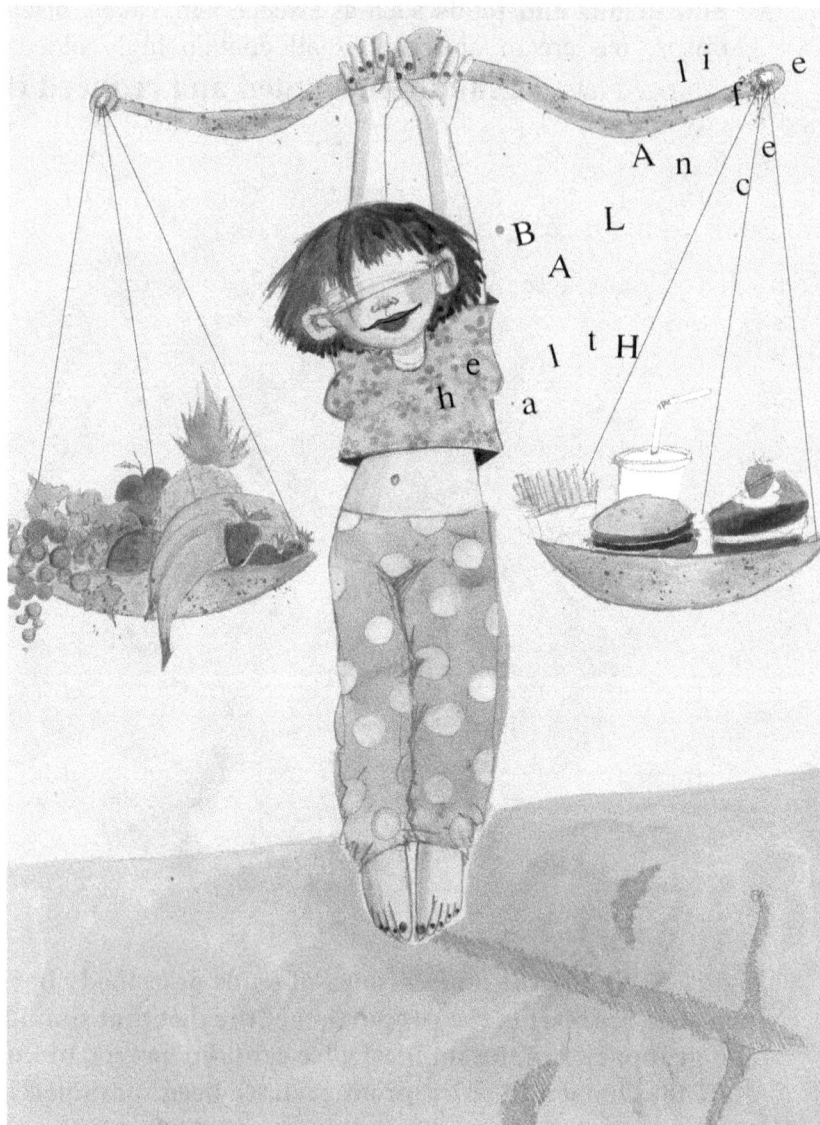

Do not beat yourself up mentally if you lapse with your diet as your new exercise regime (see Chapters 9-11) will more than compensate for the odd uncontrollable urge. Also, it has been shown that junk food rich in fat and sugar can be **addictive** just like tobacco or other drugs so **MAKE GRADUAL CHANGES**.

- **I CAN HEAR SOME OF YOU SAYING:**

- "but my diet is healthy and I am still overweight"

    or

- " I saw that television program on people inheriting a "fat gene"* and I think that I am one of those people"

    or even

- "I have a slow metabolic rate, I just look at food and the pounds go on"

GENERALLY, NONE OF THESE ARE WHOLLY TRUE AND WHAT IS HAPPENING IS THAT YOUR DAILY ACTIVITY IS NOT USING UP ENOUGH OF THE CALORIES TAKEN IN WITH YOUR FOOD

This imbalance can change rapidly at different times in your life such as following **marriage**, during **pregnancy**, as you **age** and stop participating in sport, or even as the **children grow up** or following the **death of the dog**. Similar inertia can result from **depression** and the **breakup of a marriage**, **retirement, illness, bereavement** and a **change of job**.

This decreased physical activity, for whatever reason, will result in a loss in muscle mass. Then, since the muscles are the most metabolically active (i.e. calorie-burning) tissue in the body, their loss will result in increased weight unless your food/calorie intake is reduced.

*See, for example, reference 5 for details of the so-called "fat gene".

Figure 7. Shows some of the reasons for declines in physical activity

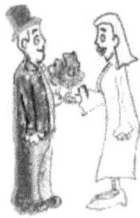

Marriage

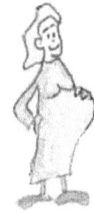

Pregnancy

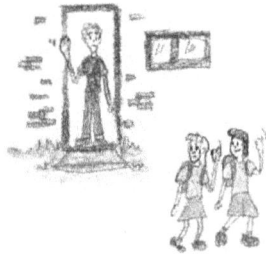

Children grown up

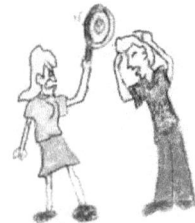

Divorce

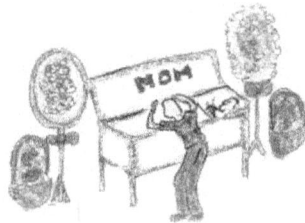

Bereavement

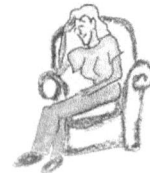

Depression

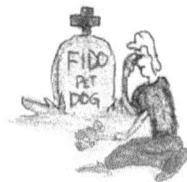

Death of dog

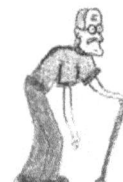

Aging

Why not sit down and tick off any of the above appropriate to you or other **REASONS THAT YOUR PHYSICAL ACTIVITY HAS DECLINED?** This may help you understand your weight gain in recent years. Of course, we lose muscle mass due to hormonal changes as we age, but again this can be compensated for by adjustments in diet or exercise regimes (see Chapters 2 and 9-11).

Finally, since we are trying to **BE REALISTIC** here, I can hear you saying that the simple healthy food options described above "will take **too much time to prepare**". It's much easier to run down to MacDonalds or the chip shop and stoke up with junk food before getting on with the more important things in life. There is no easy answer to this except to say that **FEW THINGS ARE MORE IMPORTANT IN LIFE THAN GOOD HEALTH**. Ignore this fact at your peril as father time catches up with us all but **much sooner than later** if you neglect your body.

If you simply cannot change your diet, then try eating the same things but in smaller portions. This will result in considerable weight loss and encourage you to modify your diet and eat healthier. Remember, you may not be particularly overweight but still be eating junk and have elevated levels of unhealthy fats such as dangerous types of cholesterol. These in turn will block your arteries and increase your risk of heart disease.

DAILY CALORIE REQUIREMENTS OF MEN AND WOMEN*. To generalize, the number of calories needed by women to maintain body weight is **2000 kcal** while for men it is higher at **2500 kcal**. These are very broad generalizations and will vary significantly according to your sex, age, height, weight and daily activity levels. People with lean muscular bodies who exercise regularly will need more calories than fatter people who are less active. Men also tend to need more calories than women. There are numerous tables for calculating your daily calorie requirements and your result will vary according to the table used (for example, see **www.realage.com/NutritionCenter/calorieCount.aspx** which is very useful since the calculation includes not only your height, weight, sex and level of activity but also your age). A quick calculation sometimes given is to:

For men: **multiply your weight in lbs by 14**

For women: **multiply your weight in lbs by 12**

Examples: **187 lbs (85 kilo) elderly male   = 187 x 14 = 2618 kcal**

132 lbs (60 kilo) elderly female = 132 x 12 = 1584 kcal

These results are extremely general since the calorie requirements shown are very low and only accurate for elderly people who are not very active. Increase the activity and decrease the age and much higher calorie requirements will be obtained (see also Chapter 2, page 40).

A recent report by the Scientific Advisory Committee on Nutrition (SACN), a committee of independent experts that advises the Food Standards Agency and Department of Health, has found that present calculations of calorie requirements are underestimated by approximately 16% (see reference 6). Thus, the 2000 kcal recommended for women would be 2320 kcal.

This **does not mean** that we can all go and eat an extra cheeseburger per day. This revised calculation resulted from an underestimate of the average physical activity of people in the UK, particularly for routine activities of daily living on energy expenditure. The report is only in draft form, will cause confusion and has yet to be approved.

ALWAYS REMEMBER WEIGHT GAIN OCCURS WHEN

"CALORIES EATEN EXCEED CALORIES USED BY BODY"

For example, every day eat 500 less kcal + take more exercise = weight loss

TO LOSE WEIGHT all you will have to do is reduce food intake by 500 kcal per day (3500 per week) or exercise more. Why not combine the two and cut out a mince pie, a packet of crisps or reduce food portion size (each about 250 calories less) and cycle or walk briskly for 30 min per day or for a longer time 2-3 times per week. Any combination will reduce/burn more calories.

- **BEWARE - Do not reduce food intake too quickly at the same time as you are increasing exercise or you will greatly stimulate your appetite**

BODY MASS INDEX (BMI)

Body Mass Index is a useful way of determining if you are overweight and calculating the ideal weight for your height. BMI can be calculated as follows:

BMI = your weight in kilograms divided by your height in metres squared

- **Example 1:**   woman weighing 60 kg (132 lb = 9 stone 4.3 lb) and 1.7 m (5ft 7in) tall

$$BMI = \frac{60}{1.7 \times 1.7} = \frac{60}{2.89} = 20.76$$

- **Example 2:**   man weighing 85 kilos (187 lb = 13 stone 3.4 lb) and 1.88 m (6ft 2in) tall

$$BMI = \frac{85}{1.88 \times 1.88} = \frac{85}{3.53} = 24$$

BMI Categories

- less than 18.5   =   underweight
- 18.5 to 25   =   normal weight
- 25 to 30   =   overweight
- 30 to 40   =   obese
- over 40   =   very obese

NB: Sometimes BMI can be misleading so that men with well developed muscles, such as rugby players or athletes , may have high BMIs and be classified as overweight or even obese which, of course, they are not.

TAP WATER OR BOTTLED WATER?

According to the **Drinking Water Inspectorate** (DWI, http://www.dwi.gov.uk) in 2003, 2.9 million tests of tap water were undertaken and 99.88 % passed. **This does mean that 3,480 failed**. Also, outbreaks of the diarrhoea parasite, *Cryptosporidium,* in 2006 are still fresh in the minds of many people in Wales. In 1988, the population of the

Cornish town of Camelford also drank water contaminated with excessively high levels of aluminium sulphate accidentally added to the tap water. Subsequently, on the basis of the post-mortem of just one person dying, the suggestion has been made that this incident was linked to the development of an Alzheimer's-like disease in this patient. The DWI also monitors tap water for **bacteria, pesticides, nitrates from fertilizers, and metals such as lead.** All of these substances have been reported, in a small number of tap water samples, to exceed safety levels (see details in "Water Quality in Your Region" at <u>www.dwi.gov.uk</u>).

- **SHOULD WE THEREFORE ONLY DRINK BOTTLED WATER?**

- **IT IS NOT THAT SIMPLE SINCE:**

- **There are different forms of bottled water:**

  i. Mineral Water which is natural, untreated and from a named source identified on the label. The addition of minerals is not allowed. Babies and young children should not drink mineral water due to high salt or sulphur content.

  ii. Spring Water is again from a named source shown on the label but it may have minerals added or be artificially carbonated.

  iii. Bottled Water in which the source is not identified and could be from the tap as with PepsiCo's Aquafina . Many bottled waters are just **filtered tap water** with the chlorine removed. **Crystal Spring**, for example, was produced from tap water in the basement of a London restaurant! **Flavoured Waters** should be avoided due to their content of artificial sweeteners, including aspartame and acesulphame, as well as preservatives like benzoic acid (see Chapter 5 "Additives, Preservatives and Colourants", for more details).

UNFORTUNATELY, it has been shown that bottled water of all types can be contaminated with bacteria, fungi, synthetic organic chemicals, arsenic etc (see: <u>http://www.nrdc.org/water/drinking/nbw.asp</u> for details) The latest example was in July 2007, when the Foods Standard Agency (<u>http://www.food.gov.uk/news/pressreleases/2007/jul/bottledwater</u>) alerted consumers to the risk of bacterial contamination in Hadham Naturally Pure English Spring Water which was then removed from sale.

IN ADDITION, there are reports that toxic chemicals can be absorbed from the plastic containers into the bottled water. One such toxic substance is antimony which was shown to leach very rapidly from the plastic into the water when stored for just 3 months. **The sell by dates of many bottled waters, of all 3 types, is**

often 1-2 years! Antimony could potentially be very dangerous as are other chemicals that can leach out of the plastic container. These include phalates which are released from the plastic if the bottle is filled with acidic fruit juice and are cancer forming and hormone disruptors (see Chapter 6 "The Cocktail Effect").

CONCLUSIONS, from the above, it is obvious why people are confused. The author's opinion is that it is simply not worthwhile buying bottled water of any description because:

1. There is little evidence that bottled is purer than tap water in the UK

2. Due to 1-2 year storage before drinking, dangerous chemicals could potentially leach into the water from the plastic and the environment

3. It costs too much

4. The plastic bottles are either thrown everywhere or incinerated to liberate dioxins and are an environmental disaster

5. It is simply insane to generate high levels of carbon in the manufacturing of plastic bottles and their transportation from country to country

6. Due to high levels of minerals in some bottled water, it should not be given to babies and young children and should not be used to make up baby feeds

7. Do not be afraid to ask for tap water in restaurants but remember they are entitled (would you believe) to charge you for the ice and service

THE BEST COMPROMISE IS PROBABLY TO BUY A WATER FILTRATION SYSTEM with the cheapest with a filter (Brita, Wilkinson etc) that slots into a plastic (!) reservoir. Water can be rapidly filtered and then decanted into a glass bottle and stored in the refrigerator. The filter should be changed regularly (every month) to avoid growth of bacteria trapped by the filter. Such simple filters will significantly reduce metal contaminants including lead from plumbing and aluminium from water treatment plants but are less effective against copper or fluoride. They also remove chlorine but **not** some of the harmful by-products of chlorine but these evaporate off the filtered water after storage for several hours. The best option is to install a proper water filtration system above the sink. This, however, can be expensive, but if you are concerned about possible toxic effects of fluoride added to the tap water then a portable reverse osmosis filter can be bought for about £150 and is easily fitted (**www.eastmidlandswater.co.uk**). There is a very active ongoing debate about the advantages/disadvantages of water fluoridation but even bottled water may have significant levels of fluoride. Water fluoridation is now banned in the majority of countries in Europe but still carried out in areas of the UK (see: **http://www.dwi.gov.uk/consumer/fluoridemaps.pdf** for details in your area). The author has no connection with any water filtration company.

SUMMARY FOR A HEALTHIER DIET AND WEIGHT CONTROL

• BE DETERMINED TO CHANGE
• AVOID FAD DIETS
• EAT BREAKFAST
• STOP SNACKING
• SELECT HEALTHY FOODS WITH LOWER FAT AND SALT
• GET RID OF PROCESSED FOOD FROM THE DIET
• GET ENOUGH FIBRE
• EAT AT LEAST 5 PORTIONS OF VEGETABLES OR FRUIT EACH DAY
• DRINK PLENTY OF WATER
• MAKE CHANGES GRADUALLY
• LIST REASONS FOR DECLINE IN PHYSICAL ACTIVITY

REMEMBER to change your lifestyle slowly so that your new diet and exercise regimens become a natural part of everyday living

CHAPTER 2

MORE ABOUT FOOD

HELP! WHAT AM I EATING?

Table 1 (see page 41) lists the **calorie, fat, salt and sugar** content of different types of food and will help in planning a healthier diet. It will assist in identifying those foods and snacks that are a **danger to your health** and really should be eliminated or reduced in the diet. Table 1 **also gives the fibre content** of foods as a further assistance in selecting a healthy diet (see Chapter 3 for "Facts About Fibre").

HOW TO USE TABLE 1

The colour coding in Table 1 is based upon the Food Standards Agency's **TRAFFIC LIGHT COLOURS** (see reference 7). In Table 1 these colours are converted into different shades of grey/white, as below:

DARK GREY	High Levels**	
MEDIUM GREY	Medium Levels	
LIGHT GREY/WHITE	Low Levels	Very Low Levels+

** The stars in the dark grey colour draw attention to **very high levels** of calories, fat, salt and sugar. The more stars the higher the levels.

+ The light grey/white colour is used to draw attention to those foods that are **very low in harmful substances** such as saturated fats or **very high in beneficial fibre**.

The dark grey colour indicates those foods that have an excess of harmful calories, fat, salt or sugar and which should be reduced in your diet

The medium grey colour indicates those foods that do not contain an excess of harmful calories, fat, salt or sugar but should occasionally be replaced by healthier options

The light grey/white colour indicates those foods that are low or   very low in harmful nutrients or high in beneficial fibre. The more of these foods you have the healthier your diet

A SIMPLE EXAMPLE OF HOW TO USE TABLE 1
(see page 41 for Table 1)

- Patients who have suffered heart attacks or strokes often have **high blood pressure** (hypertension) and are advised to reduce their daily intake of salt as well as to adopt a low-fat diet.

- It has, however, been calculated that **processed foods** (rather than the salt pot) may account for **75% of the daily consumption of salt**.

- It is therefore vitally important to be able to **identify those foods with high salt levels** and to eliminate them from the diet.

- Using Table 1, it is easy and very rapid to identify the high salt-containing foods just by **looking down the column labelled "Salt Grams"**.

- All foods with **high salt contents will be identified in dark grey**. For some foods, the results are not surprising as with high salt in ready meals and burgers but **salt is also present but hidden in other foods,** such as some breads, sandwiches and breakfast cereals.

- **Do take into account the amount of a particular food eaten** i.e. the number of slices of bread or ounces or grams when estimating your salt intake. The weights of each food from which levels of calories, fat etc have been calculated are given in the far left column, alongside the name of the food.

- Table 1 does not include the over 50,000 different foods found in supermarkets but includes the main groups of food so that reasonable estimates can be made. (for additional foods not in Table 1, see references 8-10).

- The same simple exercise of looking down the appropriate column and reading off the name of the food can be done for checking on calories, fat, saturated fat, fibre and sugar.

CASE STUDY -THE AUTHOR

Even the author does not completely eliminate dark grey coloured foods shown in Table 1 and he has a particular weakness for dark chocolate and chocolate biscuits. After all, **life has to be worth living,** especially when writing a book over a number of years. It is a question of controlling these urges, being aware of which foods contain harmful levels of fats, salt and sugar and only eating these **occasionally**.

The following is a guideline to the number of calories* required daily and limits on the daily consumption of fat, saturated fat, salt and sugar:

"Average" Woman** (ca. 63.5 kilo (140 lbs), 25 yr old, 5ft 4" tall, active)	"Average" Man** (ca. 73 kilo (161 lbs), 25 yr old, 5ft 8" tall, active)
Calories 2300 kcal***	Calories 3000 kcal***
Fat 70 g	Fat 95 g
Saturated fat 20 g	Saturated fat 30 g
Salt 6 g	Salt 6 g
Added sugar 50 g	Added sugar 70 g

* Each kilocalorie (kcal) = 1000 calories, and the term "kilocalorie" and "Calorie" (with large "C" often written as "Cal") are the same thing". Some articles on nutrition sometimes use calorie (small "c") to mean kcal which is confusing. In Table 1 "Calories" refers to "kcal".

** The number of calories, fats and sugar required will, of course, vary according to how much the person weighs, as well as their age and the amount of exercise taken daily (see also Chapter 1, page 31).

*** Note, the recent recalculations of calorie requirements discussed in Chapter 1, pages 31- 32.

Table 1. SHOWING CALORIE, FAT, SALT, FIBRE AND SUGAR CONTENTS OF SOME COMMON FOODS

Type of Food[1]	Calories	Fat grams (of which saturates)	Salt grams	Fibre grams	Sugar grams
FISH ▶	Most fish are low in harmful saturated fats, salt and sugar but note high saturated fats in battered fish and scampi ▼				
Cod fillet , 100g (3.5oz)	80	0.7 (0.1)[2]	0.3	0	0
Cod, Young's, battered, frozen, 1 fillet, ca.137g	271	15.6 (8)		1.7	0.5
Herring, (=kipper), Scottish hot smoked fillet, 1 typical, 80g	205	15.8 (3.8)	1.6	0	0
Lemon sole, 1 fillet 150g	125	2.3 (0.3)	0.5	0	0
Lemon sole, breaded, 1 fillet, 160g	330	14.2 (1.4)	1.7	2.2	2.9
Scottish Mackerel Tesco, 1 fillet, 100g	310	24.9 (6.7)	1.9	0	0
Mussels, ½ live pot, 140g	141	5.6 (3.5)	0.7	1.4	1.8
Prawns, Tesco, cooked and peeled, 100g	72	0.6 (0.1)	1.5	0	0
Rainbow trout, 1 x 140g	231	14.3 (3.4)	0.4	0.7	0
Salmon farmed, 1 fillet, 130g	265	17.7 (4)	0.25	0	0
Sardines, Princes, in tomato sauce, 100g	190	11.9 (3.3)	1.25	0	1.6
Sardines, Princes, in olive oil, 100g	222	13.9 (3.1)	1.25	0	0
Scampi, Young's, frozen, 100g	219	12.4 (6.5)	1.2	2.1	1.9
Seafood collection, Tesco, mussels, crab, prawns, 100g	105	2.2 (0.7)	1.05	0	0.7
Tuna chunks, sunflower oil, drained, one small can, 185g, (6.5oz)	270	12.6 (2)	0.5	0	0
MEAT/MEAT PRODUCTS ▶	Note very high calorie, saturated fat levels and salt in some mince, pies, sausages and McDonalds ▼ ▼				
Beef rump steak (fat trimmed) 200g (7oz)	307	7.2 (3)	0.3	0	0.2
Chicken mini breasts, skinned, 200g (7oz)	206	2 (0.6)	0.6	0	0
Chicken thighs – one 165g (6oz)	174	7.8 (2)	0.2	0	0
Duck, 125g (4.4oz) roasted	334	27.8 (7.8)	0.3	0	0
Lamb, Welsh, 2 chops (fat trimmed), 84g	150	6.4 (3.4)	0.3	0	0.1

Type of Food[1]	Calories	Fat grams (of which saturates)	Salt grams	Fibre grams	Sugar grams
Lamb, Welsh, leg, roasted (fat trimmed), 100g	175	8.2 (4.2)	0.4	0	0.1
Pork rump steak (fat trimmed) 200g (7oz)	273	7.4 (3)	0.3	0	0
Turkey, breast, fillet medallions, 100g	110	1.2 (0.6)	0.3	0	0
Mince, pork, 225g (8oz)	288	10.4 (4)	0.3	0	0
Mince, steak, lean 225g (8oz)	418	13.3 (6)	0.45	0	0.1
Mince, beef, 225g (8oz)	720	63 (29)***	0.35	0	0.1
Mince, lamb, 225g (8oz)	518	40 (20)***	0.35	0	0.1
Bacon, thick cut back, 2 grilled rashers, 54g	175	14.1 (4.7)	2.3	0	0
Faggots, pork, Mr. Brains, frozen, 2 ca. 188g	256	12.2 (4.8)	2.8	1.6	1.2
Pate, Tesco smooth, Brussels, 50g	164	15.9 (6.1)	1	0.8	0.4
Pate, Tesco Healthy Living, Brussels, 50g	100	7.6 (3.2)	1	1	0
Pie, pork, Melton Mowbray, small, 140g (5oz)	535	35 (13)*	1.6	0	4.2
Pie, steak and ale, deep fill, puff pastry, per 150g (5.4 oz)	344	20 (8.7)	1	2.8	1.3
Pie, steak pie, 150g (5.4 oz)	445	27 (13)*	1.5	3.8	1.7
Sausages, pork and Bramley apple, 2 grilled	386	29 (12)*	1.8	1.8	9.5
Sausages, thick pork , 2 grilled	225	13 (4.7)	2	1.7	1.1
Sausages, finest chunky Cumberland pork, 1 grilled	266	20 (7.7)	1.3	1	2.1
Sausages, beef, 2 grilled	270	18 (7.3)	1.8	0	0.5
Scotch eggs, snack, two =90g (3oz)	270	18 (5)	1.4	1.6	0
McDonalds Hamburger, 100g (3.5oz)	250	8 (3)	1.2	3	7
McDonalds Big Mac, 214g (7.5oz)	495	23 (10)*	2	5.3	8.9
McDonalds Cheeseburger, 100g (3.5oz)	300	12 (6)	1.5	3	8
McDonalds Quarter Pounder with cheese, 100g, (3.5 oz)	515	25 (12)*	1.2	4	9
McDonalds Big Tasty	840***	50 (21)***			
McDonalds Big Mac + Large Fries + Large Milk Shake!!!!!!!!	1470***	59 (21)***	3.5	12.3	92****
DAIRY PRODUCTS ▶	Note high fat levels in butter, whole milk and many cheeses ▼				
Butter, Lurpack spreadable, 10g (about one dessert spoon)	73	8 (3.7)	0.09	0	1

Type of food[1]	Calories	Fat grams (of which saturates)	Salt grams	Fibre grams	Sugar grams
Butter, Anchor spreadable, 10g	72	8 (3)	0.12	0	<1
Spread, Utterly Butterly, 10g	53	6 (1.5)	0.16	0	0.5
Spread, Flora original, 10g	53	6 (1.2)	0.1	0	<1
Spread, St Ivel extra light, 10g	19	2 (0.5)	0.1	0.13	0.14
Milk whole, 200 ml, 1 glass	128	7 (4.8)	0.2	0	9.4
Milk semi-skimmed, 200 ml	100	3.6 (2.2)	0.2	0	9.6
Milk skimmed, 200 ml	73	0.6 (0.2)	0.2	0	9.8
Milk, chocolate flavour, Superlife, 200 ml	126	1.2 (0.8)	0.25	1	20.8*
Milk Soya, organic, unsweetened, 200 ml	65	3.8 (0.6)	0	1.2	0.2
Yoghurt natural Greek style, 100g (3.5oz)	145	11 (7)*	0.3	0	6.6
Yoghurt natural, low fat, 100g (3.5oz)	65	1.5 (0.9)	0.2	0	7.2
Yoghurt Muller Light cherry, 100g	48	0.1 (0.1)	0.1	0.2	6.4
Yoghurt Muller Light strawberry, 100g	51	0.1 (0.1)	0.1	0.2	7.2
Cheese, Brie, 100g	334	28 (17)*	0.6	0	0.45
Cheese, Brie healthy, 100g	60	3.3 (2)	0.5	0	0
Cheese, Camambert, average all brands, 100g	300	24 (15.3)	2.1	0	0.6
Cheese, Cheddar extra mature, West Country Farmhouse, 100g	412	34 (23)*	1.75	0	0
Cheese, Danish Blue, 100g	350	29 (18.3)	3.7	0	0.7
Cheese, Dutch Edam, 100g	335	25 (17)**	2.6	0	0.1
Cheese, Natural Cottage, 100g	105	4.8 (2.3)	0.75	0.6	1.8
Cheese, Parmesan, grated, 100g, ca. 1 cup	431	28.6 (17.3)*	1.5	0	0.9
Cheese, Wegmans, Stilton, white with apricots, 100g	333	26.7 (20)	1.75	3.3	10
Cheese spread, Kraft Philadelphia, one tablespoon, ca. 30g	75	7.2 (4.8)	0.25	0	1
Cheese spread, Kraft Philadephia Light, 30g	47	3.5 (2.3)	0.75	0.1	1.2
Eggs, 1 egg, 55g	83	6.2 (1.8)[3]	0.1	0	0
Eggs, 2 scrambled, variable depends if use skimmed or whole milk	200 +	14+ (4+) cholesterol	0.5	0	1.4
CEREALS/CEREAL PRODUCTS – FLOUR, RICE, BREADS, BREAKFAST CEREALS ETC ▶	Note high salt levels in one slice of some bread and high salt and sugar levels in many cereals. ▼			▼	
Flour, McDougalls, self raising, 100g	315	1.4 (0.2)	0.75	3	1.3
Flour, Allinson, self raising, whole meal, 100g	325	2.2 (0.4)	0.75	9	1.9

Type of food[1]	Calories	Fat grams (of which saturates)	Salt grams	Fibre grams	Sugar grams
Pasta, Penne, white, dry, 100g	357	1.7 (0.5)	0.3	2.5	3.5
Pasta, Penne, wholemeal, dry, 100g	316	2 (0.4)	0.3	10	4
Rice, Uncle Bens, long grain, raw, 100g	344	1.25	0	1	0.5
Rice, Ambrosia, creamy rice pudding, tinned, 200g	186	3.6 (2.2)	0.5	0	16.4
Rice, Ambrosia, low fat rice pudding, tinned, 200g	166	1.6 (0.8)	0.5	0	16.4
Bagels,New York,plain white,1 bagel(85g)	216	1.6 (0.2)	0.7	2.5	5.1
Bagels, Food Doctor, highbran + seed + cranberry, 1 bagel	212	1.6 (0.34)	0.5	5.7	7.14
Bread, Kingsmill soft white, 1 slice	111	1.2 (0.1)	0.55	1.2	1.9
Bread, Kingsmill, wholemeal, 1 thick slice	100	1.7 (0.2)	0.46	2.7	1.9
Bread, Tesco, white, 1 thick slice	105	0.7 (0.1)	0.5	1.3	1.9
Bread, Tesco, organic white, 1 thick slice	110	1 (0.1)	0.5	1.4	1.4
Bread, Hovis, square cut white, 1 extra thick slice	155	1 (0)	1**	2	3
Bread, Hovis, organic, wholemeal, 1 slice	92	1.3	0.48	3.3	1.6
Bread, Nimble, white, 1 slice (ca.20g)	49	0.4	0.28	0.4	9.3?
Bread, Nimble, wholemeal, 1 slice	48	0.6 (0.1)	0.23	1.5	0.5
Bread, Warburtons, Danish lighter white, 1 slice (26g)	61	0.4 (0.2)	0.3	0.6	0.6
Bread, Mastermacher, organic sunflower seed wholemeal rye, 100g	191	3.6 (0.6)	1.25	7.9	0.7
Bread, malt loaf, Tesco, 1 x 30g slice	81	0.48 (0.24)	0.24	6.2	1.86
Bread, garlic, Tesco, 2 white baguettes, ½ baguette	300	15.9 (9.9)**	0.8	2	2
Bread, Naan, ½ naan bread	269	11 (?)	trace	1.7	40?carbs
Poppadoms, Sainsbury, plain, fried in vegetable oil, 3 = 24g	96	4.2 (?)	0	2.1	10.2 ? carbs
Croissant, Tesco Healthy Living, 1 croissant, 48g	153	4.1 (2.4)	0.5	1.6	3
Croissant, Tesco Finest, all butter, 1 croissant	330	19.4 (11.7)**	0.75	1.7	3
Cereal bars, Tesco, fruit and fibre, 1 bar, 27g	110	2.7 (1.1)	0.25	1.1	7.3
Cereal bars, Jordans, special muesli, 1 bar, 40g	151	4.6 (1.2)	trace	2.3	15.6
Cereal bars, Kellogg's, nutri-grain, choc-chip, 1 bar, 45g	179	6 (1.5)	0.2	1.5	16
Hot cross buns, Tesco Finest, white, 1 bun	205	3.2 (1.4)	0.5	2.3	13.5

Type of food[1]	Calories	Fat grams (of which saturates)	Salt grams	Fibre grams	Sugar grams
All Bran, Kellogg's, 100g	280	3.5 (0.7)	1.5	27	17
Branflakes, Tesco, 100g	326	2 (0.5)	1.3	15	22
Coco Pops, Kellogg's, 100g	387	3 (1.5)	1.15	2	36 ***
Cornflakes, Kellogg's, 100g (3.5oz)	372	0.9 (0.2)	1.8**	3	8
Cornflakes, Tesco, 100g	380	1.2 (0.4)	0.6	3	8.9
Cornflakes Crunchy Nut, Kellogg's, 100g	397	5 (0.9)	1.15	2.5	35***
Frosties, Kellogg's, 100g (3.5oz)	371	0.6 (0.1)	1.15	2	37**
Fruit and Fibre, Tesco, 100g (3.5oz)	370	6.6 (3.6)	0.75	7.7	26.5**
Oatibix, Weetabix, 2 biscuits	181	3.8 (0.6)	0.18	3.5	1.5
Special K, Kellogg's, 100g	374	1.5 (0.5)	1.15	2.5	17
Shredded Wheat, Nestle, 2 biscuits, 44g	217	3.2 (1.4)	0	5.3	6.3
Weetabix, 2 biscuits, 38g	127	0.75	0.24	3.75	4.4
Muesli, Alpen Original, 100g	359	5.8 (0.7)	0.38	7.3	22*
Muesli, Alpen no added sugar, 100g	353	5.9 (0.7)	0.43	7.7	16
Muesli, Tesco Swiss Style, 100g	359	5.3 (0.8)	0.5	7.4	21*
Porridge, Tesco, organic, 100g	360	8.1 (1.6)	0	8.5	1.5
Porridge, Scots Porridge Oats, original, 100g	356	8 (1.5)	0	9	1.1
Porridge, Ready Brek, 100g	359	8.7 (1.2)	trace	7.9	1
VEGETABLES, FRUITS AND NUTS ▶	This list is not exhaustive since most vegetables and fruit are low in calories, harmful fat, salt, and sugar as well as containing beneficial fibre ▼	▼	▼	▼	▼
Beans, fine green, organic, 100g (3.5oz)	25	0.5	0	-	2.3
Broccoli, 100g (3.5oz)	31	0.2	0	2.7	1.1
Broad beans, baby, frozen, 100g	72	0.9	0	4.6	0.9
Butter beans, raw, 100g	305	1.7 (0.2)	0	16	3.6
Carrots, 100g	36	0.3	0	2.5	7.4
Peas, frozen, 100g	77	0.25	0	5.5	4.6
Peppers, organic, 1 pepper	11	0.2	0	-	9
Potato, baking, 1 potato, ca. 175g	138	0.4	0	2.3	1.1
Salad, Tesco French style crispy, 40g	6	0.2	0	0.6	0.6
Stir-fry, Tesco vegetables, 100g	31	0.4	0	2.6	4.5
Sweetcorn, 100g	110	2.3 (0.3)	0	2.8	2.2
Tomatoes, Tesco, Italian, peeled, plum, 200g = half can	46	0.4	0	1.8	8
Apples, Granny Smith, 1 apple, ca. 133g	64	0	0	2.3	15.2[4]
Avocado, 1 ca. 145g	275	28.3 (5.9)[5]	0	4.9	0.7
Banana, 1 medium size	119	0.4 (0.1)	0	1	26[4]
Blueberries, 3 heaped tablespoons, ca.50g	25	0.2	0	1.4	5.5

Type of food[1]	Calories	Fat grams (of which saturates)	Salt grams	Fibre grams	Sugar grams
Grapes, red seedless, 10 grapes, ca. 50g	30	0	0	0.35	7.7
Mango, 250g	143	0.5	0	6.5	34.5[4]
Melon, honeydew, 1 cup, balls, 177g	64	0.2	0.1	1.4	14.4[4]
Oranges, 1 ca. 154g, edible part	59	0.2	0	2.6	13.1[4]
Pears, 1 ca. 170g	68	0.1	0	3.7	26[4]
Pumpkin seeds, Neal's Yard, organic,15g	85	6.6 (1)	trace	0.8	0.16
Sultanas, Neal's Yard, organic, per 15g	42	trace	trace	0.3	10.4[4]
Tinned prunes in fruit juice, ½ can, ca. 90g	125	0.3	0	3.5	28.6[4]
Tinned prunes in syrup, ½ can, ca. 120g	205	0.4	0	5.9	48.3**
Pineapple, 100g	44	0.2	0	1.2	10.1
Strawberries, organic, 100g (3.5oz)	27	0.1	0	1.1	6
Brazil nuts, Planters, 50g, about 12 nuts	339	34 (7.1)[5]	0	3.6	1.8
Peanuts, dry roasted, KP, 1 small bag, 50g	292	23.1 (4)[5]	1	3.3	2.6
Peanuts, original salted, KP , 1 small bag, 50g	295	24.5 (4.4)[5]	0.75	4.5	2.7
Walnuts, Planters, 50g	375	35.7 (3.5)[5]	trace	3.5	1.8
READY MEALS, PASTAS, PIZZAS, ▶ QUICHES	Note that many of these are very high in calories, fat, salt and sugar. Compare also Tesco Healthy Living Options with Tesco Finest (Finest Fat Levels*) ▼		▼	▼	▼
MOST OF THE MEALS BELOW ARE SOLD FOR EATING JUST BY ONE PERSON AND THEREFORE DATA ARE SHOWN FOR THE **WHOLE MEAL** RATHER THAN PER 100G					
Chicken tikka masala and rice, Tesco Healthy Living, 450g	480	8.6 (2.6)	1.1	3.6	13.8
Chicken tikka masala and rice, Tesco Finest, 375g	510	35.9 (13.7) **	2.4	5.7	10.5
Chicken korma and rice, Tesco Healthy Living, 450g	487	9.9 (5)	1.3	3.5	11.3
Chicken korma and rice, Tesco Finest, 500g	830 ****	45 (16.6) **	2.9	4.7	9.3
Chicken mango curry and rice, Tesco Healthy Living, 450g	495	8.1 (3.1)	1.7	4.1	20.3**
Vegetarian vegetable korma and rice, Tesco, 450g	621 **	26.4 (10.2) **	2.2	6.3	17.6
Beef and black bean sauce, Tesco Finest, 350g	336	10.9 (2.3)	3.3	5.7	16.2

Type of food[1]	Calories	Fat grams (of which saturates)	Salt grams	Fibre grams	Sugar grams
Sweet and sour chicken, Tesco Finest, 400g	560	16 (2.2)	3.2	3.4	37.8 ***
Cannelloni, beef, Tesco Finest, 400g	545	30.5 (11.6)**	2.1	4.5	11.7
Chicken with mozzarella & pancetta, Tesco Finest, 450g	830	50.2 (28.2)***	3	7.4	1
Cornbeef hash, Tesco frozen, 400g	500	17.4 (9.2)	3.6	5	0.2
Cottage pie, Tesco Healthy Living, 500g	460	13.2 (7)	1.9	5.2	2.8
Fish pie, creamy, Tesco Finest, 400g	500	26.5 (13.9)	2.1	5.3	4.4
Lasagne, Tesco Finest, 620g	850	44.6 (21)***	3.8	5	1.2
Lasagne, Tesco Healthy Living, 430g	426	11.2 (5.6)	2.3	3	1.7
Macaroni cheese, Tesco Healthy Living, 385g	420	8.9 (6)	1.7	5.8	8.9
Moussaka, lamb, Tesco Finest, 350g	510	38 (8.2)**	2	12	11.9
Pasta bake, chicken, Tesco Healthy Living, 400g	415	5.6 (2.9)	1	5.6	7.2
Pasta bake, tuna, Tesco Healthy Living, 400g	360	4.4 (1.9)	1.5	4.4	9.6
Pasta, cheese, Tesco, 400g	940***	63 (16.4)***	1.2	3.2	7.2
Pasta, tomato, Tesco, 400g	760	36 (2.8)	4.5	5.6	18
Pizza, cheese, Tesco, 395g, ½	495	17.6 (7.1)	2.8	7.5	4.5
Pizza, ham + pineapple, Tesco, 466g, ½	480	14.9 (6.5)	2.2	6.8	11.2
Pizza, pepperoni, Tesco, 398g, ½	510	18.7 (6.4)	3.1	5.6	4.6
Pizza, pizzeria, margherita, Tesco, 460g, ½	545	24.4 (12.9)**	2.2	6.2	4.8
Quiche, cheese and bacon, Tesco, 330g, ½	460	30.8 (12.4)**	1.2	2	4.8
Quiche, cheese and onion, 330g, ½	460	30.2 (12.8)**	1	1.8	5.6
Strogonoff, vegetarian, mushroom, Tesco, 450g	526	21.9 (13.2)**	1.5	5.5	4.3
SALADS, DIPS AND SANDWICHES ▶	Note high calorie, saturated fat and salt levels in some items especially sandwiches ▼	▼	▼		
Salad, chicken layered bowl, 200g	135	1 (0.2)	0.5	4	4.8
Salad, chicken and bacon, layered bowl, 200g	247	13.4 (1.2)	0.5	4	4.8
Salad, cheese layered bowl, 200g	335	26.4 (6.6)	0.7	3.2	5.8
Salad, prawn layered bowl, 200g	270	17.2 (2.5)	1.1	2.4	3.2
Salad, tuna layered bowl, 200g	274	14.2 (0.9)	0.2	2.9	3.7
Salad, creamy coleslaw and potato, 200g	450	45 (4.4)	1	3	4.3

Type of food[1]	Calories	Fat grams (of which saturates)	Salt grams	Fibre grams	Sugar grams
Dip, caramelized onion & roast garlic, ¼ pot, 50g	250	26 (3.4)	0.6	0.2	1.6
Dip, caramelized onion humous, reduced fat, ¼ pot, 50g	79	4.5 (0.5)	0.6	-	2.8
Dip, cheese and chive, ¼ pot, 50g	270	27.4 (4.2)	0.6	-	1
Dip, guacamole, ¼ pot, 50g	105	10.5 (4)	0.3	1.8	0.9
Dip, humous, ¼ pot, 50g	160	13.4 (1.4)	0.7	1.7	0.5
Dip, salsa, ¼ pot, 50g	28	1.2	0.6	0.6	2.8
Dip, sour cream & chives, ¼ pot, 50g	180	18.4 (4.2)	0.4	-	1.2
Dip, West Country Cheddar, ¼ pot, 50g	255	25.9 (4.19)	0.6	0	1.19
Make your own low fat sandwiches - see [6]					
Sandwiches, Pret a Manger, all day breakfast, malted wholegrain, 2 sandwiches	608	35.7 (8.6)**	3.54*	4.2	8
Sandwiches, cheese and chutney, with mayo, organic, malted brown, 2 sandwiches	545	29.2 (14)**	2.1	5.2	11.2
Sandwiches, cheese and onion, with mayo, brown + oatmeal, 2 sandwiches	555	33.1 (12.1)**	1.8	5.5	3.5
Sandwiches, chicken salad, malted brown, 2 sandwiches	445	20 (3.7)	1.2	6.3	4.3
Sandwiches, chicken and bacon, sub roll, white	645	29.1 (3.6)**	2	5.2	7.2
Sandwiches, ploughman's, wedge, white	605	32 (13.8)**	2.3	5.4	13.8
Sandwiches, prawn & mayo, white + oatmeal, 2 sandwiches	430	25.7	1.75	4	2.5
Sandwiches, red Cheddar and tomato, white, 2 sandwiches	490	26.6 (10.5)**	2.2	5.5	2.9
Sandwiches, roast beef, Tesco Finest, malted brown, 2 sandwiches	450	17.1 (4.6)	2.9*	ca.4.6	8.2
Sandwiches, salmon & cucumber, Tesco Healthy Living, 2 sandwiches	262	4 (0.9)	1.5	3.3	2.6
Sandwiches, smoked ham & mustard, white, 2 sandwiches	385	16.8 (3.6)	2.9*	1.9	5.9
Sandwiches, tuna-sweetcorn, malted brown, 2 sandwiches	440	21.1 (3.5)	2.5	4.4	4

Type of food[1]	Calories	Fat grams (of which saturates)	Salt grams	Fibre grams	Sugar grams
SNACKS-BISCUITS, CAKES, CHOCOLATE AND ICE-CREAM ▶	Note that many of these are very high in calories, fat, salt and sugar. These are really harmful snacks if eaten in excess daily. We all have to eat some occasionally! ▼	▼	▼		▼
Biscuits, Mcvitie's milk chocolate digestive, 4 biscuits	336	16 (8.4)**	1	2	20**
Biscuits, Mcvitie's original digestive, 4 biscuits	280	13 (6)	1	2	10
Biscuits, Mcvitie's chocolate chip cookies, 4 biscuits	332	18 (10)**	1	2.4	22.4**
Biscuits, Mcvitie's Hobnobs, 4 biscuits	268	12.4 (5.6)	1	3.2	13.6
Biscuits, Mcvitie's Hobnob flapjacks, 1 flapjack, 33g	313	14.6 (6.5)	0.5	4.7	20.5**
Biscuits, Mcvitie's Penguins, 2 biscuits	228	12.2 (7.8)*	trace	1	17.8*
Biscuits, Jammie Dodgers, 4 biscuits	332	12 (5.6)	trace	1.6	22.4**
Biscuits, Cadbury's chocolate fingers, 8 Fingers	240	12 (4.8)	trace	0.8	15.2
Biscuits, Jacob's fig rolls, 4 biscuits	252	6 (2.8)	<1	2.4	21.6**
Biscuits, Mcvitie's classic rich tea, 4 biscuits	152	5.2 (2)	<1	0.8	6.8
Biscuits, Tesco, Custard Creams, 4 biscuits	240	10.4 (6.4)	0.1	0.8	12.8
Biscuits, Cookie Coach, clotted cream shortbread fingers, 4 fingers	424*	24.2**	?	?	46.4** carbs
Biscuits, Jaffa Cakes, 4 biscuits	184	4 (2)	trace	1.2	26**
Cakes, doughnut, fresh cream, one	260	12.6 (6.4)	0.6	1.5	11.6
Cakes, cheesecake, strawberry and double cream, ¹/₅, 100g	271	13.4 (6.6)	0.2	1.6	22**
Cakes, Cupcakes, Bakin Boys, triple chocolate, one	156	9 (3)	0.1	1	12
Chocolate, Aero, 46g bar	251	14.5 (9.4)**	0.1	0.4	26.8**
Chocolate, Bounty Milk, 57g bar	267	6.8 (?)	0.14	1.2	13.6
Chocolate, Cadbury's Dairy Milk, 10 squares = 40g	220	12 (8)**	0.1	1	21**
Chocolate, Cadbury's, Dairy Milk, whole nut, 49g bar	270	17.3 (8)**	0.1	?	23.6**
Chocolate, Galaxy bar, milk chocolate, 47g bar	254	14.8 (?)	?	?	27.1 carbs
Chocolate, Kit Kat, 4 finger bar, 42g	212	11(?)	?	0	26 Carbs

Type of food[1]	Calories	Fat grams (of which saturates)	Salt grams	Fibre grams	Sugar grams
Chocolate, Maltesers, one bag, 37g	183	8.5 (?)	?	0	24 carbs
Chocolate, Mars bar, 65g bar	284	11.1(ca.6.5)	?	0	45** carbs
Chocolate, M&Ms, peanut chocolate candies, 45g bag	232	11.7 (4.7)	?	1.5	22.9**
Chocolate, Plain, Tesco, 50g (1.75oz)	259	13.5 (8.5)**	0	1.6	29.2**
Chocolate, Plain, Marks and Spencer, extra fine dark chocolate 50g	277	22.6 (13.6)**	0	6	13.5
Chocolate, Snickers, 62.5g bar	319	17.8 (ca.6.4)	0.35	1	ca.30 **
Chocolate, Twix, two fingers, 57g	284	13.9 (5.1)	0.28	0.6	27.4**
Ice-cream, cherrylicious, Tesco, 200 ml serving, about 2 scoops	240	6.8 (5.8)	trace	1	22.6**
Ice-cream, Cornish, Walls, 200 ml	166	8 (5.4)	0.26	0.2	18.4
Ice-cream, vanilla, Carte D'Or, 200 ml	240	11 (?)	?	?	29 carbs*
SNACKS-TINNED BEANS AND SPAGHETTI, CHIPS, CRISPS AND ▶ SOUPS	Note that some items are high in calories and fat but that healthier options do exist ▼ ▼				
Beans, baked and tinned, Heinz, 100g	73	0.2 (trace)	0.8	3.8	5
Beans, baked and tinned, Heinz, reduced sugar and salt, 100g	66	0.2 (trace)	0.5	3.8	3.4
Spaghetti, tinned, Heinz, 100g	60	0.3 (trace)	0.6	2.4	4
Chips, Tesco oven chips, crinkle cut, 100g (3.5oz)	140	3.9 (0.5)	0.2	1.8	<0.1
Chips, McDonald's, medium portion	340	17 (2)	0.7	4	1
Chips, Burger King, french fries, medium portion, 117g	387	20 (5)*	1.3	3	1
Crisps, Doritos, cool original, 40g pack	200	11 (1)	0.8	1.2	1.6[7]
Crisps, Hula Hoops, salt and vinegar, 34g pack	174	9.7 (0.9)	0.75	0.6	0.3[7]
Crisps, McCoy's, ridge cut, salted, 50g pack	262	16 (4.8)	1	2.1	0.2
Crisps, McCoy's, ridge cut, cheddar and onion, 50g pack	258	15.3 (4.6)	1	2	1[7]
Crisps, McCoy's, ridge cut, salt and vinegar, 50g	257	3.1 (2)[7L]	1.4	2	0.5[7]

Type of food[1]	Calories	Fat grams (of which saturates)	Salt grams	Fibre grams	Sugar grams
Crisps, Walkers, prawn cocktail, 34.5g pack	181	11.4 (0.9)	0.5	1.4	0.7[7]
Crisps, Walkers, ready salted, 34.5g pack	183	11.7 (0.9)	0.5	1.4	0.3
Crisps, Walkers, cheese and onion, 25g pack	131	8.3 (0.7)	0.32	1	0.6[7]
Soup, cream of tomato, ½ can, 300g,	169	5.7 (1.1)	1.6	1.2	15.5
Soup, chicken and sweetcorn, ½ can, 300g	127	2.7 (1.4)	1.1	2.4	5.7
Soup, pea and ham, ½ can, 300g	164	6.3 (3.9)	1.4	3.6	8
SNACKS-FISH FINGERS, KEBABS, PIES, PASTIES, RIBS, SAUSAGE ► ROLLS, AND WINGS	Not surprisingly many of these items are high in calories and fat ▼ ▼				
Fish fingers, Tesco "Free From", 3 fish fingers, 90g	180	8.1 (3.9)	0.9	0.6	trace
Kebabs, Tesco, 12 chicken tikka, pack =130g,	216	9.6 (3.6)	1.2	1.2	8.4
Pie, chicken and vegetable, each pie, 150g (5.4 oz)	390	21.8 (11.1)**	1.5	1.7	2.4
Pie, steak, 150g	445	27 (13)**	1.5	3.8	1.7
Pasty, Cornish, 150g	433	26.8 (12.7)**	1.7	5.7	3.5
Pasty, cheese, 150g	392	23.5 (11.3)**	1.7	5.8	3.4
Ribs, sticky barbecue, ½ pack, 400g	325	21.8 (9.2)**	0.7	1.9	10.5
Sausage rolls, Tesco, pack of 6, medium/large 400g, each roll 66.5g	240	16.2 (7.1)**	1	0.7	0.5
Wings, sticky barbecue chicken, ¼ pack of 500g	180	10.6 (2.8)	0.8	0.5	2.9
DRINKS-SOFT, JUICES, BED-TIME, ► COFFEE, TEA AND ALCOHOL	The items causing the main concern here are added sugar in soft and bed-time drinks and the high calories in bed-time and alcoholic drinks. ▼ ▼				
Soft drink, Coca Cola, 250 ml glass, sugar added	105	0	0	0	27[7]*
Soft drink, Diet Coca Cola, 250 ml glass	3.5	0	0	0	0[8]
Soft drink, Ribena, blackcurrant, from concentrate, 250 ml glass + added sugar	128	0	0	0	30.3*
Soft drink, Juiceburst, pomegranate, from concentrate, 250 ml + added sugar	122	<0.25	?	?	28.75*

Type of food[1]	Calories	Fat grams (of which saturates)	Salt grams	Fibre grams	Sugar grams
Soft drink, Fanta orange, 250 ml glass, added sugar	108	0	trace	0	26.3*[7]
Soft drink, lemonade, 250 ml glass, added sugar	117	0	0	0	28.5*
Soft drink, Robinsons orange barley water, diluted 45 ml in 250 ml glass	45	0	0.025	0	9
Fruit juice, apple, Sainsbury, from concentrate, 250 ml glass	117	<0.12	<0.4	<0.12	28[9]
Fruit juice, cranberry, Sainsbury, from 10% concentrate, 250 ml glass + added sugar	123	trace	trace	trace	29.8*
Fruit juice, orange, Sainsbury, 100% pure squeezed, 250 ml glass	110	0	<0.3	1	24.2[9]
Fruit juice, pineapple, Sainsbury, pure from concentrate, 250 ml glass	132	<0.12	<0.4	<0.12	31[9]
Fruit juice, pomegranate, RJA Foods, superjuice, from concentrate, 250 ml glass	110	<0.1	trace	0	26.5??
Fruit juice, tomato, Sainsbury, from concentrate, 250 ml glass	37	<0.12	2	1.7	6.7
Bed-time drink, Bournville Cocoa, Cadbury, per 4g with semi-skimmed milk	110	4.3 (2.5)	0.35	0.5	10[9]
Bed-time drink, Bournvita, Cadbury, per 12g serving	140	3.7(?)	?	?	20[9] carbs
Bed-time drink, instant hot chocolate, Tesco, 30g in water	125	3 (2.6)	0.5	0.6	19.1
Bed-time drink, Horlicks original, per 20g with 200 ml semi-skimmed milk	186	4.6 (2.6)	0.5	0.7	19.6
Bed-time drink, Ovaltine original, per 25g with semi-skimmed milk	187	3.8 (2.1)	0.4	0.6	21.71 *
Bed-time drink, Ovaltine original light, per 25g in water	90	1.5 (0.9)	0.25	0.75	14
Coffee, black, brewed/instant, 240 ml cup	12/6	0	trace	0	0
Coffee, cappuccino, Starbucks, with skimmed milk, 240 ml cup	52	0	0.17	0	6.4
Coffee, cappuccino, Starbucks, with whole milk, 240 ml cup	84	4.4 (2.8)	0.16	0	6
Coffee, espresso, Starbucks, 30 ml single	5	0	0	0	0
Coffee, espresso, Starbucks, 30 ml single shot + dollop whipped cream	110	9 (6)*	0.02	0	2
Coffee, latte, Starbucks, with skimmed milk, 240 ml cup	84	0	0.29	0	10

Type of food[1]	Calories	Fat grams (of which saturates)	Salt grams	Fibre grams	Sugar grams
Coffee, latte, Starbucks, with whole milk, 240 ml cup	136	7 (4.4)	0.26	0	9.6
Coffee-mate, Nestle, per 6.5g teaspoon	36	2.2 (2.2) [10]	0.1	0	0.6
Teas, ordinary brands, no milk or sugar, 240 ml cup	0	0	0	0	0
Teas, ordinary brands, with 30 ml semi-skimmed milk and 5g (1 teaspoon) sugar	34	0.5 (0.3)	trace	0	5
Alcohol, beer, bitter, 1 pint (568 ml)	182	0	trace	0	20 carbs
Alcohol, beer, Budweiser, 1 pint	183	0	trace	0	0
Alcohol, beer, Guiness, 1 pint	170	0	trace	0	8.5 carbs
Alcohol, beer, lager, Stella, 1 pint	229	0	trace	0	16 carbs
Alcohol, champagne, 120 ml glass	91	0	trace	0	1.7 carbs
Alcohol, gin, 40%, double, 50 ml	112	0	0	0	0
Alcohol, vodka, 40%, double, 50 ml	110	0	0	0	0
Alcohol, white wine, 120 ml glass	89	0	trace	0	3.6 carbs
Alcohol, whiskey, 40%, double, 50 ml	107	0	0	0	0
Alcohol, wine red, Burgundy, 120 ml glass	104	0	trace	0	4.4 carbs
DRESSINGS, PICKLES, SAUCES, GRAVIES, SPREADS ► AND JAMS	Many items are high in calories and salt but healthier options are available ▼ ▼				
Dressing, Real Mayonnaise, Hellmann's, per 20g serving	145	15.8 (1.3)	0.3	0	0.3
Dressing, Light Mayonnaise, Hellmann's, per 20g	59	6 (0.6)	0.46	0	0.4
Dressing, Salad Cream, Heinz, per 20g	66	5.4 (0.6)	0.5	trace	3.5
Dressing, fat-free vinaigrette, Hellmann's, per 20 ml	47	0	0.18	trace	2.2
Dressing, French vinaigrette, Tesco Finest, 20 ml	92	8 (0.8)	0.3	0.1	1.1
Dressing, Italian, Newman's Own, per 20g	109	12 (?)	0.4	?	1 carbs

Type of food[1]	Calories	Fat grams (of which saturates)	Salt grams	Fibre grams	Sugar grams
Pickle, original pickle, Branston, 1 tablespoon, 15g	16	trace	0.6	0.2	3.6
Pickle, original Picalli, Tesco, 15g	12	trace	0.3	0.2	2.4
Pickle, olives in brine, whole green, 15g	20	2 (0.4)	0.8	3.1	trace
Pickle onions in sweet vinegar, Sainsbury, excess vinegar dried, per 15g	5	trace	0.26	1.1	0.9
Sauce, tomato ketchup, Heinz, per 20g	20	trace	0.6	0.1	4.7
Sauce, brown, HP original, per 20g	24	trace	0.5	0.3	4.5
Sauce, pasta, slow roasted garlic and chilli, Seeds of Change, organic, 100g	73	4.5 (1.3)	1.4	1	7.3
Sauce, pasta, tomato and basil, Seeds of Change, organic, 100g	59	2 (0.4)	0.8	0.8	7.8
Sauce, pasta, traditional bolognaise, Seeds Of Change, organic,100g	58	1.2 (0.3)	1	0.8	8.9
Sauce cooking, Indian, Korma, Sherwoods, gluten –free, 100g	136	7.8 (4.4)	1	2.2	7.7
Sauce cooking, Indian, Rogan Josh, Sherwoods, 100g	71	3.8 (0.3)	1	3.5	4.7
Sauce cooking, Indian, Tikka Masala, Sherwoods, 100g	116	7.7 (3.3)	1.6	1.6	6
Sauce cooking, Chinese, black bean and red pepper, Sherwoods, 100g	62	1.4 (0.2)	1.7	1.2	5.9
Sauce cooking, Chinese, sweet and sour, Sherwoods, 100g	105	0.5 (trace)	0.9	0.8	17.9
Gravy, Oxo beef, each cube, 5.9g	16	0.27 (0.13)	2.5	trace	0.15
Gravy, Bisto original, 4 level teaspoons = 1 serving + water	9	trace	0.8	trace	0.2
Gravy, Tesco beefy drink/stock, like Bovril, 1 teaspoon	24	trace	1.4	?	trace
Spread, honey, Sainsbury, pre-set blended, 1 tablespoon, 15g	51	trace	trace	trace	13
Spread, Marmite, 4g	37	trace	0.5	0.1	trace
Spread, peanut butter, smooth, with salt, 1 tablespoon = 15g	90	7.8 (1.5)	0.19	0.9	1.17
Jam, apricot spread, Weight Watchers, 20g	23	trace	trace	0.13	5.3
Jam, blackcurrant, reduced sugar, Sainsbury, per teaspoon	29	<0.1	<0.1	0.2	5.9

Type of food[1]	Calories	Fat grams (of which saturates)	Salt grams	Fibre grams	Sugar grams
Jam, marmalade, Frank Cooper's Oxford original, coarse cut, 20g serving	54	0	0.05	0.2	11.9
Jam, raspberry, Robertsons, 20g	49	trace	<0.1	0.3	11.9
Jam, strawberry conserve, Tesco Finest, 20g	50	trace	trace	0.2	12

Remember, stars in dark grey boxes indicate very high levels of calories, fat, salt or sugar. Often, calories, fat etc are given per 100g of food item but servings actually eaten, as with cheese, are much less than this.

1. Unless otherwise indicated, the data for many food items were taken from Tesco supermarkets.

2. Whenever possible, not only fat but also saturated fat levels are given in brackets. Saturated fats raise bad cholesterol in the blood and can lead to heart disease and other health problems (see Chapter 3 "Fats – the Good, the Bad and the Ugly").

3. Eggs are packed with protein, vitamins and minerals and have been called a superfood. The yolk, however, does have high cholesterol levels but one egg a day is unlikely to affect cholesterol level in the blood and increase heart disease (see reference 11).

4. Many fruits such as apples, bananas, mangoes, and pears, have a high sugar content but these natural sugars (called fructose) in fruit and vegetables are beneficial and different to sugar (sucrose) added to our food. Fructose is broken down slowly by the body and does not cause a sudden increase in blood sugar. In contrast, sucrose added to food causes a sudden rapid increase in blood sugar (sucrose is rapidly broken down to glucose=blood sugar) and overworks the pancreas to release insulin. Too many sudden increases in blood glucose from sucrose can stress the pancreas and may potentially lead to diabetes as well as to the conversion of the excess glucose to fat.

5. Avocados and nuts contain high levels of fat but most of this fat is monosaturated which is "good" fat and this will help reduce cholesterol.

6. See "Top tips for a healthier lunchbox" at:
www.food.gov.uk/news/newsarchive/2004/sep/lunchbox

7. These foods may contain saccharin, colourings, preservatives, stabilizers, monosodium glutamate, and/or flavourings etc. Generally, the crisps just with salt added are free of these additives. 7L= lower fat or "light" crisps are now available in many flavours.

8. Items with no added sugar but with artificial sweeteners (aspartame), flavourings, colourings, citric and phosphoric acids etc.

9. These have no added sugar and contain only natural sugar from the fruit-see 4 above.

10. Contains hydrogenated vegetable oils.

CHANGES IN DIET WITH AGE

A FACT OF LIFE! As you age, your metabolism slows down, you have less energy and so you need fewer calories. Unless you eat fewer calories or become more active, you will slowly gain weight and gradually fat will accumulate to eventually form a bulging stomach, backside, legs, arms and face which will result in becoming overweight and eventually possibly obesity too. These changes are particularly marked by an increase in waist measurement and in the size of clothes worn-the so-called "**middle age spread**". These changes are not inevitable as explained in detail in reference 12.

REALISE THAT FAT AND WEIGHT WILL ACCUMULATE WHEN:

"CALORIES EATEN EXCEED CALORIES USED BY BODY"

There are **TWO OPTIONS** to avoid weight gain with age:

1. **Reduce calorie intake** by gradually changing your diet such as switching to skimmed milk and avoiding high fat snacks (see Chapter 11, Table 2).

2. **Increase calories burnt** by slowly increasing the amount or frequency of exercise. This will not only burn the excess calories but also increase your muscular mass and metabolic rate. **MOST IMPORTANT TOO** is that age-related muscle wasting (Sarcopenia) will also be avoided and the ability to live independently will be retained longer (see Chapter 11, pages 217-220).

The reduced metabolism with age results from the loss of muscle mass and an increase in fat deposits. Muscles burn calories more actively than fat so any exercise to strengthen the muscles will also raise the metabolic rate. Unfortunately, since women have less muscular mass than men the reduction in the metabolic rate with age in women is more rapid than in men. **Women are therefore more prone than men to gain weight with age.**

Therefore, the calorific excesses some women inflict on their bodies, in particular, by drinking pints of lager, will probably be reflected by more rapid weight gain in women than in men.

Other dietary modifications with age. All the advice given above in this chapter about healthy eating should continue to be followed i.e.:

Table 2. Summary of Dietary Advice

1. Eat breakfast

2. Avoid processed food and unhealthy snacks

3. Eat less saturated fats and trans fats

4. Avoid foods with too much salt added

5. Eat plenty of fruit and vegetables

6. Have a enough fibre and water each day

7. Read and understand food labels

IN ADDITION, other changes gradually occur as we age that will affect our nutrition:

- Retirement may restrict the money available for food

- Death of, or separation from, partner may result in depression and poorly prepared food

- Senses such as sight, taste and smell of food will diminish and reduce interest in food

- Our ability to absorb certain key nutrients may be reduced sometimes as a result of medicines taken

- Constipation may be common due a reduction in saliva production and slower movements of food through the gut

- Neglect of the teeth and oral hygiene may result in inclusion of softer and more processed rather than fresh food in the diet

- **IT ALL SOUNDS VERY DEPRESSING** but remember the 7 points listed about diet (above, Table 2) as well as the following advice in Figure 1 and Table 3 (below) and sensible nutrition can then be maintained

Figure 1. Summary points for maintaining healthy nutrition with aging[a]

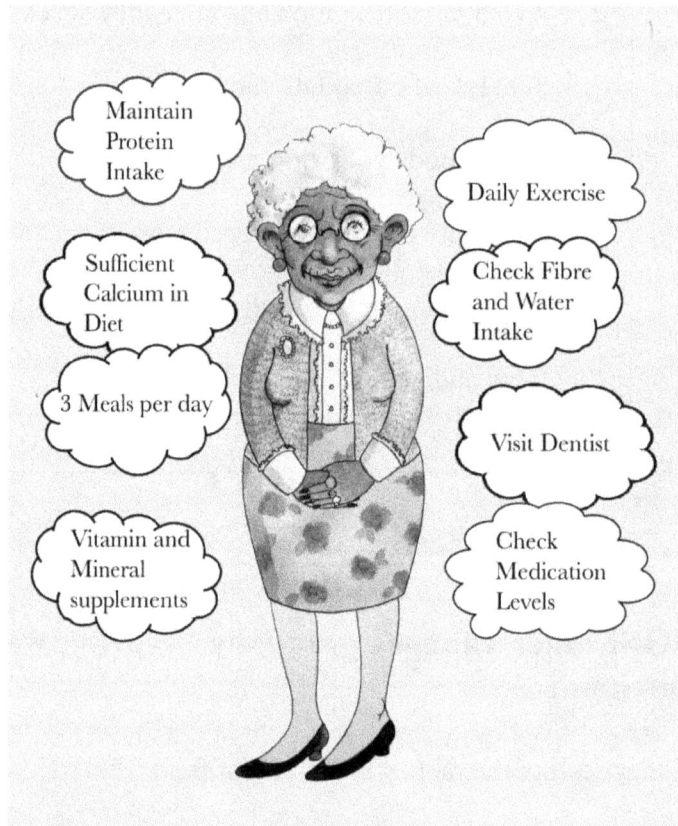

Table 3. More Details of Points in Figure 1. (above)

1. Maintain regular daily exercise to reduce depression and stimulate the appetite, to meet friends, and to maintain muscular tone and healthy bones.
2. Eat three regular meals per day.
3. Vary choice of food. Ensure that protein levels are high by eating sufficient lean meat, fish, low fat dairy products, beans and peas, wholemeal bread and, if possible, a whey protein drink.
4. To maintain healthy bones, make sure that sufficient sources of calcium are included in the diet. Natural calcium sources are low fat dairy products, sardines, salmon, green vegetables etc.
5. Older people with poor diets or with illnesses may require vitamin and mineral supplements. Be aware that "Recommended Daily Allowances" have been calculated for younger people. Consult your doctor as supplements may interact with medicines.
6. Reduce likelihood of constipation by increasing amount of natural high fibre foods and drinking about 8 glasses of water, juice or soup daily.
7. Regularly check with doctor that medicines taken are both necessary and at the correct dose. Also, check on possible interactions of medication with absorption of essential nutrients.
8. Visit dentist regularly to maintain healthy teeth and gums.

a. See, also, Chapters 7 and 8 "Vitamins, Minerals and Supplements Dilemma"

SUMMARY

Follow the above advice together with regular exercise and you will be revitalised and always remember to:

• BE DETERMINED TO CHANGE
• AVOID FAD DIETS
• EAT BREAKFAST
• STOP SNACKING
• SELECT HEALTHY FOODS WITH LOWER FAT AND SALT
• GET RID OF PROCESSED FOOD FROM THE DIET
• GET ENOUGH FIBRE
• EAT AT LEAST 5 PORTIONS OF VEGETABLES OR FRUIT EACH DAY
• DRINK PLENTY OF WATER
• MAKE CHANGES GRADUALLY
• LIST REASONS FOR DECLINE IN PHYSICAL ACTIVITY

Change your lifestyle slowly so that your new diet and exercise regimens become a natural part of everyday living

CHAPTER 3

More Facts About Food, Fat, Fibre And Fad Diets

FATS – THE GOOD, THE BAD AND THE UGLY

- **"Fats are bad for you".** We have all heard this so many times. Fats are reported to cause cancer, obesity and heart disease.

- **Fats, however, are essential because they:**

  i   make up the walls of cells and tissues
  ii.   are an energy source
  iii.   form precursors of some hormones
  iv.   are involved in absorption of vitamins A, D, E, and K

- **Confused?** No wonder! The reason for the poor understanding about fats has arisen due to the fact that there are several different types of fat in our food, namely:

  i.   **monounsaturated fats**
  ii.   **polyunsaturated fats**
  iii. **saturated fats**
  iv. **trans fatty acids (=hydrogenated vegetable oils)**

These 4 names for the different types of fats are the ones found on **food labels.**

It is therefore important to understand that some fats are good for us while others are bad and associated with heart disease, cancer, etc.

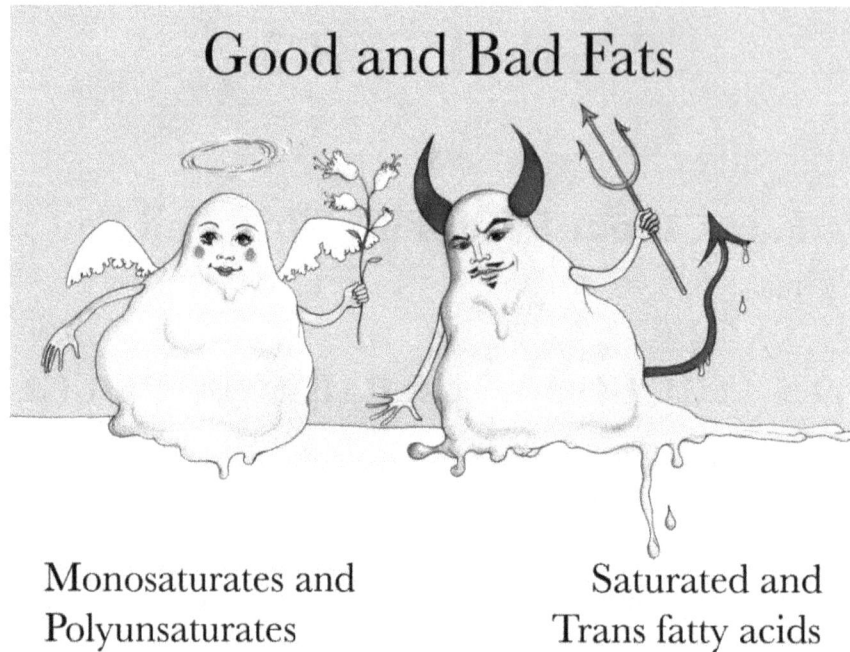

Good and Bad Fats

Monosaturates and
Polyunsaturates

Saturated and
Trans fatty acids

Good fats **are the unsaturated monounsaturates and polyunsaturates.** These are found mainly in vegetable oils and margarines made from these, as well as in oily fish like salmon, mackerel, sardines and pilchards (see, Table 1, below).

Bad fats **are the saturated and the trans fatty acids**. Saturated fats are present in full-fat dairy products, fatty meats, sausages, burgers, pies, biscuits etc. Trans fats are found in food naturally in small amounts. Most trans fats originate in the diet through "processing" by heating vegetable oils together with hydrogen. This process turns the vegetable oils semi-solid and these trans or "hydrogenated" vegetable oils are then marketed as margarines and used in biscuits, cakes, fried foods and take-way meals (see Table 1, below).

Why are some fats good and others bad? This is because the type of fat in the diet can **influence the levels of cholesterol in the blood.** High cholesterol levels are associated with increased risk of heart disease or even strokes.

You should remember 2 facts:

1. The bad fats, i.e. the saturated and trans fatty acids, **raise** the levels of cholesterol in the blood and hence increase the risk of heart disease.

2. The good fats, i.e. the monounsaturates and polyunsaturates, **reduce** the levels of harmful cholesterol in the blood and hence decrease the risk of heart disease.

Foods containing these different types of fats are summarized in Table 1:

Table 1. Showing the Distribution of Common Fats in the Diet

Type of Fat	Effect on Cholesterol Levels in Blood	Main Food Source
Monounsaturated	Lowers bad cholesterol	Olive, canola and peanut oils, most seeds and nuts (except coconuts), and avocados.
Polyunsaturated	Lowers bad cholesterol	Sunflower, corn, soybean oils or soft margarines[a] made from these oils, oily fish such as salmon, mackerel, sardines, pilchards, trout.
Saturated	Raises bad cholesterol	Full fat dairy products such as cheese, butter, whole milk and ice cream[b], coconut and palm oils, animal fats especially red meats and poultry skin, shrimps, lard, dripping, cakes, biscuits and most savoury snacks and chocolate[c].
Trans Fatty Acids = Hydrogenated Vegetable Oils	Raises bad cholesterol	Solid or semi-solid margarines, some cakes, biscuits and savoury snacks as well as many deep fried foods such as chips, doughnuts, onion rings[d,e].

a. **Check the label of soft margarine** and confirm that it is free of trans fats (often labelled "hydrogenated vegetable oils" to confuse everyone) and is non-hydrogenated.

b. Skimmed milk and lower fat ice cream or some frozen yoghurts are much better.

c. It is clearly impossible to cut out all of these completely from the diet. Depending on your weight, and with moderation and exercise, some of these can still be eaten occasionally but not to excess. **Just be aware and beware of excesses** and check for dangerous trans fats.

d. These especially and c. (above) are the key foods to check in your diet as they may contain high levels of artery clogging trans fats. **Marks and Spencer has actually banned trans fats while Sainsbury's, Tesco, Co-op, Asda, and Iceland are removing from their shelves their own brand foods containing trans fats which are hydrogenated vegetable oils** (oils exposed to hydrogen to harden them at room temperature). Also, good news is that Mars, Jammie Dodgers, Wagon Wheels and McVitie's biscuits no longer contain hydrogenated oils. **Beware since some of Lidl's foods still contain these.**

e. Recently, it was reported (see reference 13) that in the UK because food companies have removed trans fats from their foods that these heart-blocking substances are well below levels causing health hazards. Huge progress has therefore been made **BUT action is still needed with food from cafes, fish bars, canteens, hospitals etc that are still using hydrogenated vegetable oils (trans fats) in food preparation.**

FINAL CONCLUSION ABOUT FATS. The bad saturated and trans fats should be reduced in the diet as this will significantly lower your risk of heart disease. Table 1 (above) is simply a guide showing which foods contain the different types of fats so that you can reduce/eliminate them from the diet. **Again modify your diet a little at a time and you will see your cholesterol levels fall as well as your excess weight.** Adopt a healthier diet as outlined above and try some regular exercise as outlined in Chapters 9-11.

FACTS ABOUT FIBRE

- **Dietary fibre** is only found in plant and not animal products. Fibre occurs in two forms, namely, **insoluble and soluble fibre**.

- **Insoluble fibre** forms the structural support of plants, may pass straight through the gut with only minimal digestion, and helps to increase the activity of the intestine in getting rid of waste products from digestion .

- **Soluble fibre** originates from the contents of the plant cells, can be partially broken down in the gut, and absorbs water and increases the volume of faeces for ease of expulsion.

- Most fruit and vegetables contain a mixture of insoluble and soluble fibre.

- **Plant foods with high fibre levels have not been highly processed** and have not had their outer layers (seed coats etc) – which contain fibre, vitamins and minerals – removed; this removal occurs with most rice and wheat so that it is gleaming white and more attractive to the shopper.

- **Table 2 lists the fibre content of some common foods.** A balanced diet should contain about 20-25 grams of fibre per day from a mixture of fruit and vegetables (at least five per day) and high fibre breakfast cereals.

Table 2 Showing the Fibre Content of Some Common Foods[a]

Higher Levels of Fibre[b]	Lower Levels of Fibre[c]
Whole Meal Bread and Rolls	White Bread and Rolls
Whole Meal Pastas*	White Pastas**
Brown Rice	White Rice
All-Bran/Bran Flakes*	Puffed Wheat/Sugar Puffs
Weetabix*	Corn Flakes/Crunchy Nut
Shredded Wheat*	Rice Krispies, Coco Pops
Porridge Oats, Muesli	Cheerios
Baked Beans*, Peas*, Cabbage, Carrots, Spinach, Broccoli, Potatoes in skins	Salads, Tomatoes, Skinned Potatoes, Cucumber, Peppers, Celery**, Radishes
Sweetcorn	Mushrooms, Onions
Apple with skin, Pears, Avocado, Figs*, Dates, Raspberries*, Blueberries*, Blackberries*, Prunes*, Apricots, Oranges, Raisins and Dried Fruit* Bananas, Mangoes,	Strawberries, Grapes, Pineapples, Melons
Peanuts, Almonds* Coconuts*	Brazil Nuts, Sunflower Seeds
Yoghurts with Cereals and Berries (see which above)	Most Fruit Drinks, Plain Yoghurt

a. This Table is just a rough guide based on an average serving (100 gram or 3.5 oz) of the foods listed.

b. "High" is anything above 1.5-2 gm of fibre per serving.

c. "Low" is anything below 1.5 gm of fibre per serving.

*   These foods are very high in fibre.

** All fruits and vegetables contain some beneficial fibre. White pasta also has significant levels of fibre.

BENEFICIAL EFFECTS OF FIBRE. Health professionals commonly claim that there are many beneficial effects of sufficient fibre in the diet including reductions in:

Constipation
Diverticulitis
Irritable bowel syndrome
Cancer of colon
High cholesterol
Heart disease
Diabetes
Obesity
Gallstones

Controversy, however, does exists about the benefits of fibre. Some scientists challenge the assumption that fibre helps to prevent the above diseases.

Scientists often disagree even if the proof is beyond doubt. Unfortunately, the resulting debate once released in the media does nothing except **to confuse the public** as to what exactly they should eat. People then tend to shrug and continue with their bad habits having justified this to themselves since **"even the experts disagree"**. The inconsistent opinions over the value of fibre (and many other dietary components) often originate from the type of experimental analysis undertaken. Thus, questionnaires may be used in which people fail to make accurate returns. Alternatively, the time scale of the study may be too short and not take account of the fact that many diseases, such as cancers, may take 10-20 years or even longer to develop.

THE IMPORTANT MESSAGE ABOUT FIBRE is that it does help to keep the gut healthy by **preventing constipation** and possibly also irritable bowel syndrome, as well as the other conditions listed above. Evidence indicates that fibre is beneficial in **preventing cancer of the colon**, perhaps by speeding the expulsion or dilution of harmful toxins in the gut, or by providing anti-cancer chemicals (antioxidants, see

Chapter 8) linked to the fibre from the fruit and vegetables eaten. Fibre may also **reduce cholesterol levels**, and thus the incidence of heart disease, by binding and assisting in cholesterol excretion from the body. Fibre also slows down the rate at which glucose is absorbed from the food and prevents rapid fluctuations in blood sugar and may therefore **help to prevent and control diabetes.** Including sufficient high fibre foods in the diet may also **help control weight problems** by reducing hunger.

FINAL COMMENT AND WARNING. Adequate fibre is essential throughout life but is particularly important in **elderly people** who often have high levels of constipation. Each day in the diet include :

- Breakfast cereals with high fibre or porridge (see choice in Chapter 2 and Table 1 and Table 2 of present Chapter)

- Wholemeal bread

- Brown rice

- 5 or 6 or more portions of fruit and vegetables (peas and various types of beans have high fibre contents)

- See Table 2 of present Chapter for choice of main high fibre foods

- Drink sufficient water, milk, herbal teas, or soup to avoid dehydration with about 6-8 glasses sufficient

- Do not sprinkle pure fibre supplements on your food as these may bind iron, calcium and zinc in your gut which will be lost down the toilet

FAD OR TRENDY DIETS

COMMENTS ABOUT THE ATKINS AND GI DIETS

ATKINS DIET

Much has been written about this diet and for the overweight person it must sound like **advice from heaven** to try a diet advocating eating almost unlimited meat, eggs, cheese, butter, sausages and bacon whilst discouraging bread, rice and fruit! This diet is basically high in fat and protein but contains very little carbohydrate – no more than 20 grams per day. On the basis of this diet, Atkins published two books entitled "Dr.Atkins Diet Revolution" in 1972 and "Dr.Atkins New Diet Revolution " in 1999, and these together sold about 25 million copies. The reason for this success was undoubtedly because of the huge media hype by the New York Times, CBS and numerous follow-up stories that appeared throughout the USA and eventually in the UK and elsewhere. In addition, many people who tried the Atkins diet reported rapid losses in weight and described him as "a great man". The fat in the Atkins diet was believed to reduce the appetite and stop cravings for carbohydrate.

Figure 1. Showing some of the high fat foods recommended by Atkins

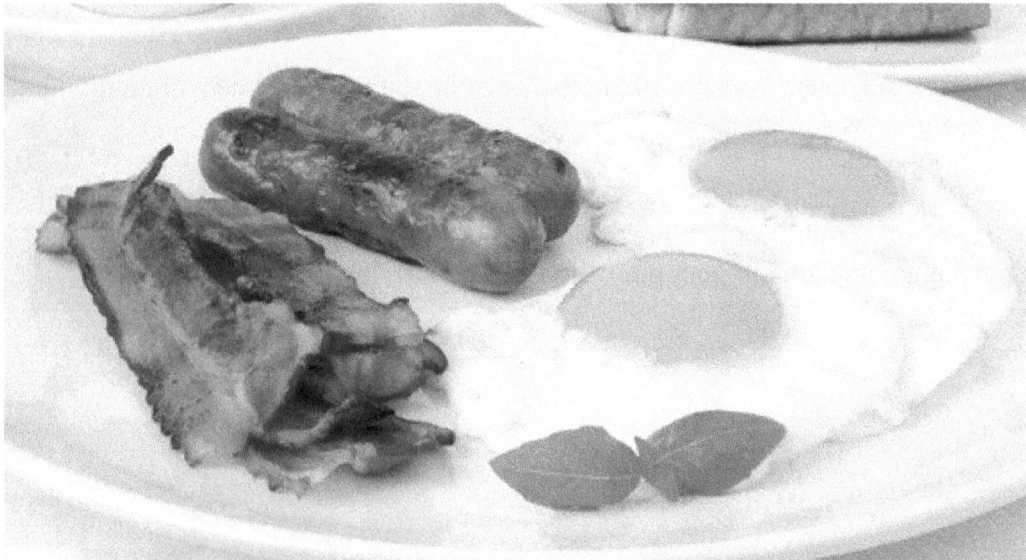

The problem with the Atkins diet is that it is extremely high in animal fats. It also limits the intake of fresh fruit and vegetables and whole grain breads that are the cornerstone of healthy nutrition advocated by the majority of the medical profession. Hence, the "eat five or more servings of fruit and vegetables daily" advised everywhere now.

Common sense should tell us that diets high in animal fat and low in fruit and vegetables would lack essential vitamins and minerals and potentially result in high cholesterol levels in the blood (see, however, "**Final Conclusions on Atkins**", below). Thus, the Atkins diet potentially may increase the risk of cancer, heart disease and osteoporosis (resulting in brittle bones), as well as limiting the intake of beneficial antioxidants from fruit and vegetables (see Chapters 7, 8).

These are the reasons that so **many organizations have condemned the Atkins diet** and described it variously as "negligent" and " a massive health risk"(Medical Research Council; British Nutrition Foundation, 2003), and a "serious threat to health" (American Medical Association's Council on Food and Nutrition, submission to US Select Committee,1973) (see reference 14).

BUT IT SEEMS TO WORK for rapid weight loss and this is why so many people have tried it. Unfortunately, the Atkins Diet has been shown to work for a few months but **after one year it has been reported to be less effective than simple low fat diets**. In addition, many people find it difficult to maintain the Atkins diet and drop out. Maybe this is the reason that more people have not been harmed by the extreme nature of the Atkins diet.

FINAL CONCLUSION ON ATKINS. More recently, much has been made of a few studies seemingly supporting the Atkins diet. One example, in 2007, showed that Atkins was effective for weight–loss in 311 women and even after one year had no adverse effects on cholesterol or blood pressure levels (see reference 15). Nobody knows, however, what the potential harmful long-term effects of the Atkins diet are on health. These few studies have to be balanced against the many hundred of reports showing the value of high intakes of fresh fruit, vegetables and whole grains in a balanced diet together with exercise, as described in Chapters 1 and 2 of this book. We all know how conservative the medical profession can be and how people are fed up with contrary advice given by so-called health and diet experts. **The scientific evidence, however, for using the Atkins diet is limited so be safe and follow the advice given in Chapters 1, 2 (above)** and there will be no need for any stressful new fad diets.

GI DIET

Do you really have time to embark on yet another new trendy diet designed to make money for the authors?

The GI diet basically classifies different carbohydrate-containing foods according to their **effect on blood glucose (sugar) levels** once they are digested in the gut. After digestion, glucose is released into the blood from different foods at varying rates. Thus, some foods are rapidly digested and cause **swift rises in blood glucose and have a high GI index**. Other foods are digested slowly and cause only **gradual rises in blood glucose and have a low GI index**.

Foods are often classified as having high, medium or low GI values; glucose itself has a maximum GI of 100. Food charts are available giving the GI values of different foods.

The idea of classifying foods by their GI index is that those with a high GI index will raise blood sugar rapidly so that you will feel tired, lacking in energy and hungry within a short time of eating them. In contrast, those with a low GI index raise blood sugar slowly and provide energy supplies longer so that hunger is delayed and less snacking is likely to occur.

ADVANTAGES OF THE GI DIET are that it has generally had a good reception from health professionals since eating low GI foods helps to prevent rapid fluctuations in blood sugar and may reduce the risk of Type 2 diabetes (non-insulin dependent). In addition, the GI diet may increase levels of "good" cholesterol (HDL cholesterol) in the blood and reduce the incidence of heart problems.

DISADVANTAGES OF THE GI DIET are that some foods do not seem to fit into a healthy lifestyle. Thus, crisps, milk chocolate and salted peanuts are included in the low GI category while Branflakes, Cornflakes and water melon have high GI values. This can all get very confusing. In addition, since different foods are eaten together at a meal, it may be difficult to calculate the GI index of the whole meal. In the real world, most of us do not have the time to calculate or remember GI values or the calorie contents of each meal. What we need is to develop a healthy lifestyle **for the rest of our lives**, realize generally which foods are good or bad, and take plenty of exercise as a norm.

FINAL CONCLUSION ON GI DIETS. Providing that foods with low GI values but high fat levels (salted peanuts, crisps etc) are limited then the GI diet should do no harm and some weight loss can be expected (see reference 16a). Such GI diets will, however, require some considerable menu planning with little advantage over the healthy principles described earlier in this present chapter.

Summary

1. Some fats are good for us while others are bad and associated with heart disease and cancer. Good fats are the **unsaturated monounsaturates and polyunsaturates** found mainly in vegetable oils and margarines made from these, as well as in oily fish like salmon, mackerel, sardines and pilchards (see, Table 1). Bad fats are **the saturated and the trans fatty acids**. Saturated fats are present in full-fat dairy products, fatty meats, sausages, burgers, pies, biscuits etc. Most trans fats originate in the diet through "processing" by heating vegetable oils together with hydrogen to form trans or "hydrogenated" vegetable oils and are then marketed as margarines and used in biscuits, cakes, fried foods and take-away meals.

2. There are many beneficial effects of sufficient fibre (i.e. 20-25 grams daily) in the diet including reductions in constipation, cancer of the colon, cholesterol levels and heart disease, and it may also help to prevent and control diabetes and weight problems.

3. Avoid fad diets such as Atkins and GI and follow the advice in Chapters 2-3 to control and reduce weight. Since weight control can be problematic joining together with others can reinforce maintenance of a healthy diet and exercise regimen.

Chapter 4

IS OUR FOOD SAFE?

Are Pesticide Residues Present In Our Food?

Are Organic Foods Safer?

> If you just want to know which foods contain the highest and lowest rates of pesticide residue contamination then go to pages 87 - 90 for a summary of "safe" foods

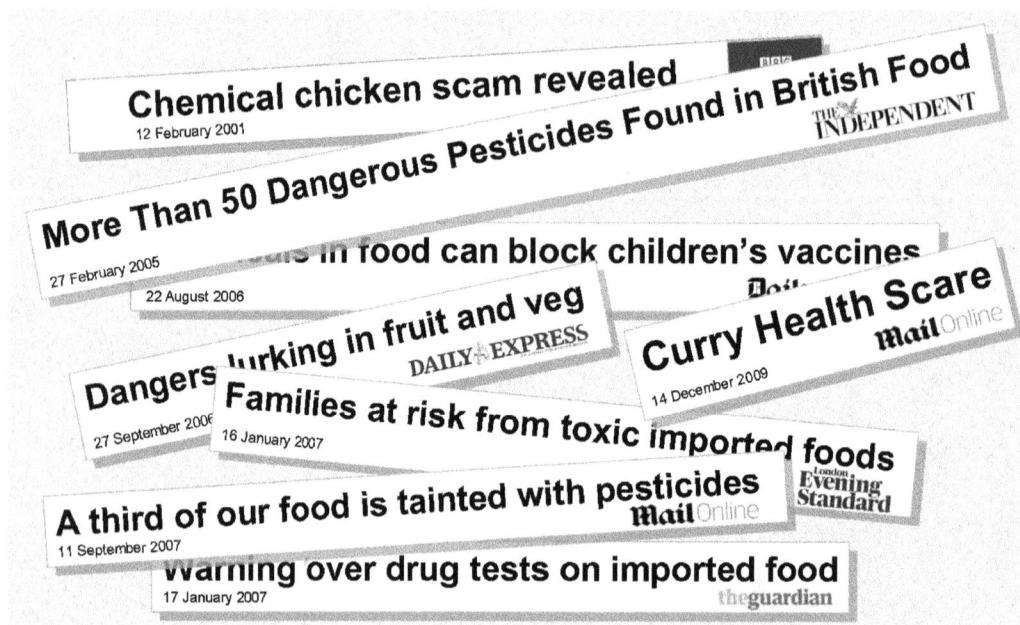

Chemical chicken scam revealed
12 February 2001

More Than 50 Dangerous Pesticides Found in British Food
THE INDEPENDENT
27 February 2005

...als in food can block children's vaccines
22 August 2006

Dangers lurking in fruit and veg
DAILY EXPRESS
27 September 200?

Curry Health Scare
Mail Online
14 December 2009

Families at risk from toxic imported foods
16 January 2007
London Evening Standard

A third of our food is tainted with pesticides
Mail Online
11 September 2007

Warning over drug tests on imported food
17 January 2007
theguardian

As far as our food is concerned, most people are suffering from **"expert opinion overload"**. Almost daily, there are articles in the press and on the radio and television talking about food quality and safety. Recent headlines are shown above.

In addition, a large number of UK organizations, set up for monitoring the safety and quality of our food, seem to be publishing reports almost daily. Thus, we have:

- The Department of Health
- The Food Standards Agency
- The Pesticides Safety Directorate
- The Pesticides Residues Committee
- The Soil Association
- The Food Commission
- The Advisory Committee on Pesticides
- The Committee on Mutagenicity of Chemicals in Food, Consumer Products and the Environment
- The Pesticide Action Network
- The British Nutrition Foundation
- The World Wildlife Fund etc, etc.

Unfortunately, as far as food safety is concerned, the opinions of the experts, the stories in the press and the reports from the above organizations are often contradictory. The end result is **CONFUSION** which:

MAY REDUCE PUBLIC TRUST IN FOOD SAFETY IN TERMS OF BOTH CHEMICAL POLLUTION AND HYGIENE

- This chapter is mainly concerned with the safety of our food from chemical residues resulting from the use of chemicals to control pests.

- Subjects such as the nutritional value of food produced by intensive conventional farming and the role of vitamins and supplements are dealt with in Chapters 7 and 8.

PUBLIC CONCERN OVER FOOD SAFETY

- A study, during June/July 2006 in the USA by Michigan State University's Food Safety Policy Centre, of over 1,014 people showed that 70% are concerned about pesticide and chemical residues while about 50% are concerned about antibiotics/hormones and additives/preservatives in food (see reference 16b).

- In the UK, public trust in food safety has been eroded following the BSE (early 1990s) and Foot and Mouth (2001) outbreaks, as well as by concern over Genetically Modified (GM) foods (1999), the Sudan I scare in Worcester Sauce (2005) and, more recently, Bird Flu and the mass slaughter of turkeys (2007).

- Previously, over 25% of the UK public believed that food is becoming more risky with particular concern over additives (see reference 17). In a European survey, concerns about pesticide levels in food were rated at the top end of the so-called "worry scale" (see reference 18). Despite reassurances about food safety, a recent UK poll showed that 59% of people interviewed were still worried about contamination of food and drink with pesticides (see reference 19).

- The public, however, does have an increase in trust for the **Food Standards Agency (FSA)** although only 34 % would consult the FSA for information on food safety and 26% for healthy eating **(www.food.gov.uk/).**

- It is obvious that many people are **TOTALLY FED-UP AND CONFUSED** with the constant and inconsistent expert and media advice about food safety and have little idea as to what to believe. The situation is bad enough to have been the butt of jokes on the Terry Wogan Radio 2 show.

- How often do you hear the comment "If you listened to the experts **you wouldn't eat anything"?** Understandably, people may find it difficult to know what to do to avoid the exposure to harmful chemicals in their food.

- Regarding the chemical contamination of food, sometimes, **the appropriate scientific study has not been undertaken** or, if it has, the results have been analysed variably by different organisations. Thus, expert agreement regarding pesticide safety levels may differ significantly.

To ordinary people, the fact that **scientific opinion can disagree widely,** even over the same set of experimental results, is surprising. One good example is the debate between the UK's Pesticide Residues Committee and scientists at the University of Liverpool **over levels of risk from pesticide residues in food** (see reference 20).

In the light of the contradictory and incomplete evidence about the potential harm of chemical pesticides, let us briefly look at some of the important issues of pesticide safety in food and arrive at an unbiased conclusion as to the **safest and most sensible ways of feeding our families.**

WHAT ARE THE FACTS?

Figure 1. Showing the origin of chemical residues in our food

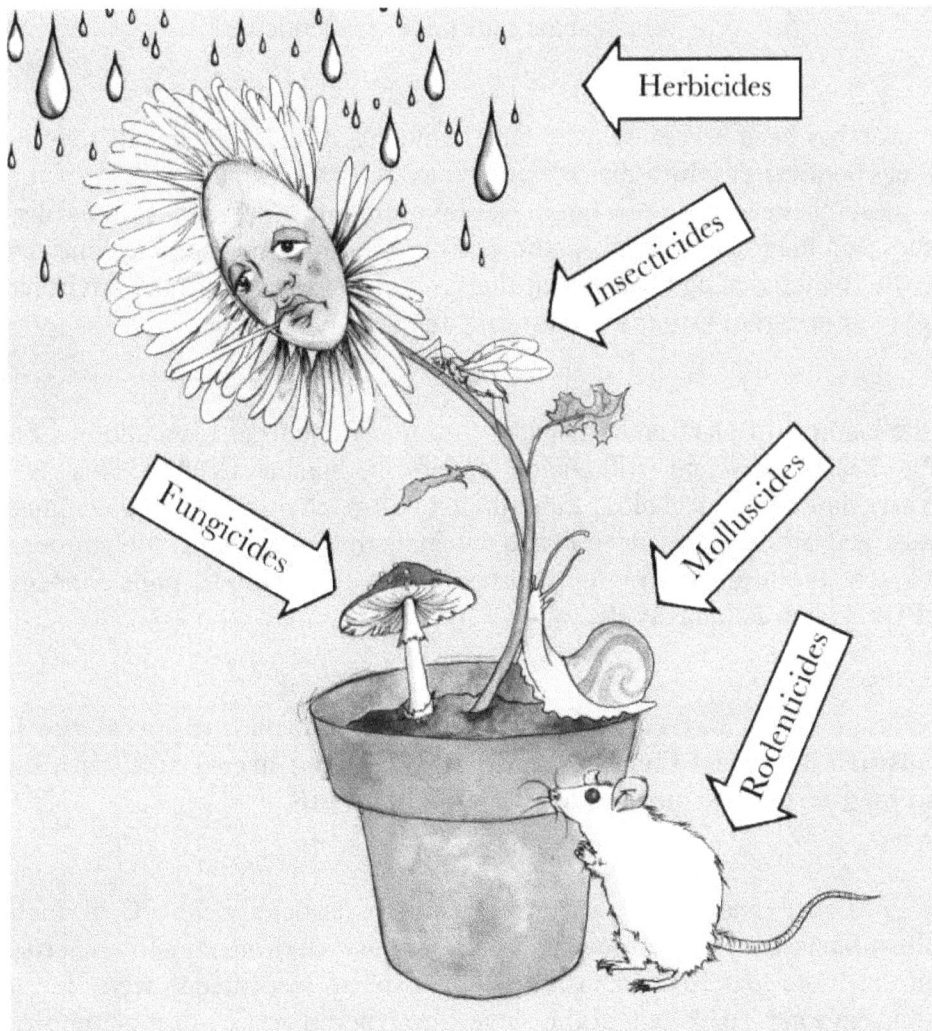

Pesticides are groups of chemicals used to control pests attacking our food crops. The results of the use of these pesticides are not entirely bad and it has been estimated that without the use of artificial nitrogen fertilizers, the World's available fertile land could only support about 60% of the present population (see reference 21). However, with the incidences of some diseases, such as cancers and allergies, increasing at alarming rates, it is time to rectify the environmental damage caused by excessive and poorly controlled use of chemical pesticides. With this aim as a priority, scientists are developing integrated pest management (IPM) programmes, minimising the use of chemicals and reducing the impact on natural animal and plant populations and human health (see references 22, 23).

These pests and the pesticides used (see Figure 1, above) to combat them include:

i. **insects** - insecticide chemicals
ii. **fungal diseases** - fungicides
iii. **weeds** – herbicides
iv. **slugs and snails** – molluscicides
v. **rats and mice** – rodenticides

After the crop has been harvested, very small amounts of these chemicals may remain in the food as **chemical residues** that are consumed by both humans and farmed animals. Many of these chemicals are not rapidly eliminated from the body as they dissolve in fatty tissues and then **accumulate in the body** over some considerable time. Examples are DDT, PCBs, dioxins and aldrin that due to their persistence in the environment are often termed **"Persistent Organic Pollutants or POPS".**

Despite the banning of DDT and other POPS in many countries (Stockholm Convention on POPs, 2001), they are still being found in human tissues. This is due to **bioconcentration** in food chains, through long-term environmental contamination of soils, water and air by pesticide use and by industrial and incineration processes. **As humans are at the top of many foodchains then we may ingest high concentrations of these POPS from fish, meat etc.**

These residual POPs may cause breast and other cancers, suppress the immune system, disturb hormonal functions and pollute human breast milk with unknown short and long-term consequences for babies and infants.

Recently developed and widely used replacement pesticides for POPS include the **organophosphates and carbamates**. These are less environmentally persistent than POPS but are more toxic to humans. Organophosphate insecticides were developed in Germany in the early 1930s but, at the same time, the potential of organophosphates as nerve gases was recognized by the Nazis. They subsequently developed organophosphate nerve gases that are often referred to as:

"Weapons of Mass Destruction"

The effects of exposure to organophosphates and carbamates are similar and include **hormonal disturbances, as well as nervous, behavioural, psychiatric and muscular disorders** such as those experienced by some Gulf War Veterans. Carbamates and organophosphates inhibit the messenger molecule, acetylcholinesterase, between nerve cells, thus preventing nervous transmission and leading to paralysis and even death. Some organophosphates are stored in fatty tissues and cleared slowly from the body. This increases the chances of **enhanced toxicity by the interaction between two or more organophosphates** or with other chemical pollutants. This process is the so-called :

"COCKTAIL EFFECT"

The importance of the cocktail effect is controversial but potentially extremely important and is discussed in detail in Chapter 6.

HOW ARE THE LEVELS OF PESTICIDES MONITORED IN OUR FOOD?

Pesticide residues were previously monitored and regulated in our food from 1977 to 2000 by a Government committee. Since 2000, this function has been taken over by an "independent" organization called the **Pesticide Residues Committee (PRC)**. Membership of the PRC, however, is still influenced by Government Ministers and Senior Civil Servants.

The PRC analyses about 4,000 food samples every year for a wide range of pesticides and the results are published four times per year. The types of food monitored are varied from year to year. The detailed reports can be read at **www.pesticides.gov.uk** . The PRC advises the Government as well as the **Food Standards Agency** (FSA, **www.food.gov.uk**/). The FSA is an "independent" Government Department "to protect the public's health and consumer interests in relation to food". The FSA was set up by the Government following the BSE crisis in the UK.

Reports (2005 to 2009) by the PRC on the pesticide residues in food and drink **concluded that the large range of conventionally-produced foods tested were safe** since:

- in about 70% of tested samples no residues were present

- in the remaining 30% of samples with residues, levels of contamination were below statutory safety limits

Despite these PRC findings, **the public still has deep concerns about food safety** (see above and at **www.foodproductiondaily.com/news**) and the PRC findings have been challenged by many organizations and individuals. One such organization is **Pesticide Action Network, UK** (PAN UK, an "independent, non-profit organization, promoting healthy food, agriculture and an environment") which in 2005 produced its own **"Alternative Pesticide Residues Report"** based on the results of the PRC reports of 2000 to 2005 in which the pesticide residues of common foods were analysed (see reference 24).

There are particular worries about the possible effects of pesticide residues in food on the delicate and rapidly growing bodies of babies and young children. In 1996, the USA National Academy of Science confirmed that any health risks of such chemicals would be magnified in the young (see details in Chapter 6, "The Cocktail Effect").

Useful reference for latest reports on food safety is:
www.foodproductiondaily.com/news

The Best and Worst Foods for Pesticide Content are Shown in Tables 1 to 3, below

NB. These Tables are taken from data in the Pesticide Residues Committee (PRC) reports of 2005-2009. In Tables 1 and 2, testing on pears, peaches, nectarines, apples (commonly eaten unpeeled) and also, for some reason, papaya, grapefruits, bananas, oranges, pineapples, lemons, citrus fruits, mangoes, melons, pineapples and probably kiwi, as well as root vegetables was carried out **WITHOUT PEELING or TRIMMING**. Thus, the contamination rates for most of this latter unpeeled produce are not included in Tables 1 and 2 since we do not eat bananas, pineapples etc with their skins on! Furthermore, much evidence shows that peeling/trimming, together with washing and cooking (see references 25-27), removes most of the pesticide contamination. This is confirmed in Tables 1 and 2 since tinned pineapples and mandarins (with peels removed) as well as shelled peas have very low contamination rates in contrast to the unpeeled fruits (90%+ contamination) and peas with pods (60%+). The USA Environmental Protection Agency (EPA) believes that the majority of pesticide residues are in the skins of fruits and vegetables and, in contrast to the UK FSA, very sensibly recommends peeling and washing all produce.

Table 1. FRUITS LISTED WITH HIGHEST AND LOWEST PESTICIDE CONTAMINATION RATES

Fruit Tested[1]	Number of Samples Tested	Percentage of Samples with Pesticides	Results with Organic Samples[2]
Strawberries	92	86-94	6 tested 0+
Apricots	50	84	4 tested 0+
Pears[3] unpeeled	181	78-97	3 tested 1+
Peaches and Nectarines[3] unpeeled	130	76-93	2 tested 0+
Apples unpeeled [3]	346	74-94	15 tested 0+
Grapes[4]	306	70-97	5 tested 0+
Raspberries	36	58	0
Blackberries	36	58	0
Cherries	46	48	0
Pomegranates	37	46	0
Nuts	64	42	3 tested 1+
Plums	72	37	3 tested 0+
Kiwi fruit [3?]	90	26-65	6 tested 0+
Avocados	21	24	3 tested 0+
Orange juice[3]	68	18	4 tested 0+
Mandarins (tinned)	18	17	0
Dried fruit [5]	48	17	4 tested 0+
Lychees	16	12.5	0
Papaya [3]	32	unpeeled	0
Grapefruits[3]	18	unpeeled	0
Bananas [3]	44	unpeeled	4 tested 0+
Oranges[3]	156	unpeeled	3 tested 0+
Pineapples [3]	47	unpeeled	1 tested 0+
Lemons[3]	33	unpeeled	2 tested 0+
Mixed citrus Fruits[3,6]	72	unpeeled	0
Melon [3]	96	unpeeled	0
Mangoes	48	unpeeled	0
Apple juice[3]	371	7.5	0
Blueberries	49	6	2 tested 0+

Olives	69	**6**	1 tested 0+
Peaches (tinned[3])	48	**4**	1 tested 0+
Pineapples (tinned[3])	18	**0**	0

More than 50% samples contaminated

20 to 49% samples contaminated

Less than 20% samples contaminated

1. Data for these fruits are taken from the Pesticides Residues Committee (PRC) reports of 2000 to 2009.

2. With organic samples, "0" means no organic samples tested while "0+" means none tested had residues.

3. NB: Many of these fruits were over 75-100% contaminated but they were tested **without peeling,** including pears, peaches, apples, papaya, oranges, grapefruits, lemons, bananas, apples, mangoes, melons, pineapples, and probably kiwi too(?). Evidence on page 78 indicates that most pesticide is removed by peeling. The fact that **whole** pineapples and peaches have high rates of pesticide residues, while tinned pineapples and peaches have much lower levels, indicates that most residues are in the skins of the unpeeled fruits.

4. Grapes are particularly high in multiple pesticide residues as they are often attacked by insect and fungal pests and have to be sprayed frequently.

5. Dried fruits are from grapes and include currants, sultanas and raisins.

6. Includes satsumas, clementines, mandarins and tangerines.

- **Note in Table 1 that most organic fruit samples are free of pesticides**

Table 2. VEGETABLES/SALADS LISTED WITH HIGHEST AND LOWEST PESTICIDE CONTAMINATION RATES

Vegetable/Salad Tested [1]	Number of Samples Tested	Percentage of Samples with Pesticides	Results with Organic Samples[2]
Baby salad [3] (bagged)	72	74	2 tested 1+
Cucumber (unpeeled)	74	69-89	22 tested 2+
Peas fresh[4] (edible pods)	46	61	5 tested 0+
Courgettes (unpeeled)	42	55-77	6 tested 0+
Rice (mixed)	70	50	2 tested 0+
Raddishes	18	50	0
Potato chips[5]	48	48	0
Spinach	101	46-55	5 tested 2+
Potato crisps[5]	132	45	3 tested 0+
Tomatoes (fresh) [4]	142	43-85[6]	2 tested 0+
Beans (green + speciality)[7]	143	38-75[6]	4 tested 0+
Potatoes [8] (unpeeled)	496	27-64[6]	18 tested 1+
Lettuce	253	26-91[6]	6 tested 0+
Aubergines	71	23-39	0
Okra	47	17	0
Peppers	178	15-61[6]	0
Turnips	36	14	1 tested 1+
Beetroot	7	14	11 tested 0+
Celery	107	13-52[6]	17 tested 0+
Pulses	84	13	4 tested 1+
Parsnips[9]	82	unpeeled	15 tested 0+
Carrots	89	unpeeled	7 tested 0+
Sweet potatoes	47	unpeeled	0
Brussel sprouts	18	Not trimmed	0
Yams	46	unpeeled	0
Onions (bulb)	14	unpeeled	9 tested 0+
Salad onions	24	unpeeled	0
Garlic	24	unpeeled	2 tested 1+

Cabbage	91	**Not trimmed**	5 tested 0+
Mushrooms	155	**9**	4 tested 1+
Peas (shelled[4] fresh & frozen)	35	**6**	1 tested 0+
Leeks	67	**5-13**	5 tested 0+
Fennel	48	**4**	2 tested 0+
Broccoli	48	**4**	3 tested 0+
Pumpkin	39	**3**	9 tested 0+
Asparagus	95	**1**	0
Cauliflower	33	**0**	3 tested 0+
Tomatoes (tinned) [4]	48	**0**	3 tested 0+
Swede	36	**0**	3 tested 0+
Corn on cob	61	**0**	0
Corn/baby	23	**0**	1 tested 0+
Marrows	59	**0**	0
Baked beans	72	**0**	5 tested 0+
Soup (vegetable)	72	**0**	2 tested 0+
Sunflour and Pumpkin seeds	48	**0**	0

More than 50% samples contaminated

20 to 49% samples contaminated

Less than 20% samples contaminated

1. Data for these vegetables/salads are from the Pesticides Residues Committee (PRC) reports of 2000 to 2009.

2. With organic samples, "0" means no organic samples tested while "0+" means none tested had residues.

3. Baby salad in bags is particularly high in numbers of samples contaminated with pesticides. In addition, more than 17 samples had more than one chemical residue.

4. The fact that peas with pods and tomatoes with skins have higher pesticide rates than shelled peas and tinned tomatoes is additional evidence that the skins of fruit and vegetables protect underlying flesh from contamination.

5. High pesticide residues in potato crisps and chips are of concern and very surprising since peels containing much of the contamination are removed prior to crisp and chip production. This elevated level of pesticides in chips and crisps probably arises during cooking since the oil used is constantly refiltered and reused. Thus, since many pesticides dissolve in fats and oil, any residues in the potatoes will gradually leach out during cooking and concentrate in the oil as it is used time and time again. High levels of pesticides will then be transferred back to the chips via the excess oil sticking to them during cooking.

6. The huge variability in contamination rates from 26 to 91% for lettuce and other foods probably results from samples tested derived from plants grown at different times of the year, or obtained from different suppliers/countries, or may be due to improvements in analytical techniques from one year to the next. Note that some vegetables are classified with "Low" (light grey) or "Medium" (medium grey) contamination rates although the upper range of their contamination rates would place them in the "High" or "Medium" ranges eg. Peppers-15 (low) to 61% (high).

7. Green beans, in particular, have fewer samples with residues than the speciality beans (long beans and soy beans).

8. Potato samples include main crop and new potatoes. During growing, potatoes are sometimes sprayed 19 times per season and 90 pesticides have been registered for use on potatoes of which only about 50% can be detected in the laboratory.

9. Root vegetables and cabbage/Brussel sprouts have not been peeled or trimmed so data for these is not included in Table 2.

- **Note in Table 2 that most organic vegetable samples are free of pesticides**

Table 3. OTHER FOODS LISTED WITH HIGHEST AND LOWEST PESTICIDE CONTAMINATION RATES[1]

Food Tested [1]	Number of Samples Tested	Percentage of Samples with Pesticides	Results with Organic Samples[2]
FISH [3]			
Salmon (farmed)	63	98	3 tested 2+
Trout (farmed)	45	67	0
Salmon (fresh)	35	60	0
Salmon (tinned)	156	24	0
Mackerel	7	14	0
Fish (deep water)	24	8	0
Trout (fresh)	6	0	0
Fish (take away)	48	0	0
Tuna (tinned)	120	0	0
Shellfish [4]	84	0	0
Prawns	48	0	0
MEAT/MEAT PRODUCTS[5]			
Lamb(New Zealand) [6]	14	29	0
Lamb (mainly UK)	97	14	6 tested 0+
Liver	96	2	0
Beef	192	1	3 tested 0+
Sausages	144	1	0
Bacon	54	0	1 tested 0+
Burgers	72	0	0
Chicken	60	0	2 tested 0+
Duck	36	0	0
Kidneys	59	0	0
Liver	71	0	0
Meats (tinned)	144	0	0
Pate (meat)	72	0	1 tested 0+
Turkey	107	0	0
DAIRY PRODUCE [7]			
Butter	120	24	4 tested 0+
Soya milk	60	8	6 tested 0+

Cream	189	**1**	1 tested 0+
Cheese (all sorts)	72	**0**	2 tested 0+
Eggs	132	**0**	12 tested 0+
Fromage frais	13	**0**	0
Low fat spreads	96	**0**	2 tested 0+
Milk (whole fat, semi-skimmed and goats)	298	**0**	65 tested 0+
Yoghurt	107	**0**	11 tested 0+
CEREALS/ CEREAL PRODUCTS			
Rye	34	**91**	0
Bran	119	**88**	12 tested 0+
Oats	34	**85**	0
Flour (wheat)	72	**72**	6 tested 0+
Bread (all types)	143	**72**	17 tested 0+
Cereal bars	96	**68**	2 tested 2+
Rice	168	**59.5**	3 tested 0+
Breakfast Cereals	144	**29**	3 tested 0+
Popcorn	29	**24**	3 tested 0+
Noodles (wheat and rice)	48	**19**	2 tested 0+
Rice cakes	48	**6**	11 tested 0+
Pizza	48	**4**	0
Pasta	144	**1**	12 tested 0+
BABY (INFANT) FOODS			
Infant food (cereal)	202	**8**	71 tested 1+
Infant food (fruit and vegetable)	72	**3**	32 tested 0+
Infant food (meat, fish, cheese)	263	**3**	93 tested 0+
Infant formula	72	**0**	2 tested 0+
DRINKS			
Wine	72	**56**	0
Beer	48	**31**[8]	0
Tea	96	**12.5**	4 tested 0+
Coffee	108	**0**	0
Water (bottled)	50	**0**	0

MISCELLANEOUS			
Herbs	51	53	0
Peanut butter	24	21	1 tested 0+
Chocolate (white)	48	12.5	5 tested 0+
Honey	72	0	6 tested 0+
Marmalade	48	0	2 tested 0+
Mayonnaise	38	0	0

More than 50% samples contaminated

20 to 49% samples contaminated

Less than 20% samples contaminated

1. Data for these foods are from the PRC reports of 2000 to 2006. Results from more recent 2008-9 reports are similar to those in Table 3.

2. With organic samples "0+" means no samples with residues while "0+" means none tested had residues.

3. Some fish, including tuna, marlin, swordfish and shark, accumulate relatively high levels of heavy metals and pregnant women should avoid these (see, " Mercury levels in fish", page 89).

4. Shellfish includes mussels, oysters, whelks and scallops but not crabs, lobsters and prawns.

5. The results for meat/meat products are for contaminating pesticides but not for artificial hormones and antibiotics, which are both banned in the EU, but often given to animals outside the EU to stimulate growth (see page 89).

6. The origin of pesticides in New Zealand lamb is as a result of persistent organochlorine (eg. DDT) contamination of the environment from past use.

7. Dairy produce should be safe from pesticides, artificial hormones contamination and antibiotics in the UK.

8. With beer DO NOT PANIC!! Pesticides in beer come from the hops but levels are very low (see reference 28).

- ## Note, with only two exceptions, that all organic samples are free of pesticides

OVERALL SUMMARY FROM TABLES 1-3 OF FOODS WITH HIGHEST AND LOWEST PESTICIDE CONTAMINATION RATES

IMPORTANT

COPY THIS LIST AND ATTACH TO NOTICEBOARD OR FRIDGE AS A REMINDER

FRUITS

Lowest rates
↓

- All fruits with peel or skins, such as citrus fruits, bananas, mangoes, pineapples, melons, apples etc, probably have the lowest rates of pesticide contamination **AFTER THE PEEL/SKIN IS REMOVED**.

Highest rates
↓

- In contrast, many "soft" fruits, such as grapes, strawberries, apricots, raspberries, cherries, plums, and peaches as well as unpeeled apples and pears, have the highest rates of pesticide contamination. Most of these are not peeled before eating and pesticides probably bind to the skins.

- Organic fruit is expensive so give priority to organic soft fruit or apples and pears if you eat the skin. Unfortunately, organic soft fruit is expensive so wash non-organic soft fruit (uncut to avoid loss of vitamins) for 30sec to 5 min.

VEGETABLES/SALADS

Lowest rates

↓

- All vegetables that are peeled/podded before eating, such as peas, peeled potatoes, tinned/peeled tomatoes, mushrooms, turnips, parsnips, onions, leeks, carrots, swedes, corn, broad beans, baked beans, etc, probably have the lowest rates of pesticide contamination.

These have low rates too!

↓

- Some items with no peel also have low contamination rates, including cabbage, okra, fennel, broccoli, asparagus, cauliflower, and marrows.

Highest rates

↓

- In contrast, items with no peel or unpeeled before use, such as bagged salad, fresh lettuce, celery, aubergines, peas with edible pods, green beans, salad onions as well as unpeeled potatoes, fresh tomatoes, cucumber, peppers and courgettes, have the highest rates of pesticide contamination.

- Organic vegetables are more expensive and often unavailable so always wash and/or trim all non-organic and unpeeled vegetables and salads. **Always buy organic potatoes which are relatively cheap and available.**

- Beware bought chips and crisps since these may have high pesticide rates from contaminated cooking oil. Make your own chips if you must.

OTHER FOODS

| Lowest rates |
↓

- Generally, fish and shellfish (except fresh and farmed salmon, and farmed trout), all meats (except New Zealand Lamb), dairy products, pizzas, pastas, baby foods, tea, coffee, bottled water, chocolate, honey, marmalade, and mayonnaise, have the lowest rates of pesticide contamination.

Highest rates
↓

- In contrast, cereals and cereal products, such as wheat flour, rye, bran, oats, rice, bread, cereal bars, and breakfast cereals, have high rates of pesticide contamination.

- Organic foods are more expensive so **IT IS MOST IMPORTANT TO BUY ORGANIC BREAD, PORRIDGE, FLOUR AND CEREAL BARS.**

Mercury levels in fish
↓

- Many fish also contain traces of mercury so that children under 16 as well as pregnant women and women planning pregnancy should avoid shark, marlin and swordfish and limit themselves to two fresh tuna steaks per week. Tinned tuna is safer. Mercury may affect the nervous system of the unborn baby and young children. Cod, haddock and plaice are fine.

Antibiotics in meat
↓

- Although meats and dairy produce have low rates of pesticide contamination, antibiotics are sometimes added to animal feeds outside the EU and these may contaminate imported foods. It is better to buy UK produce if you are certain of the origin. Organic meat and dairy produce is readily available but expensive. Marks and Spencer and Sainsbury's specialise in quality meats and poultry and sometimes are as cheap as other higher volume supermarkets.

OVERALL SUMMARY AND WHICH ORGANIC FOODS ARE MOST IMPORTANT TO BUY

1. Generally, fruits and vegetables once skinned, peeled, shelled or trimmed will probably have low pesticide contamination levels so organic is unnecessary.

2. Most soft fruits (but not blueberries) have high pesticide levels so wash thoroughly (uncut). Organic grapes and strawberries are available but expensive.

3. Always buy organic apples/pears or peel before eating.

4. Many vegetables, including lettuce, celery, and tomatoes as well as aubergines, peas with edible pods, green beans, and salad onions have high pesticide rates but buying organic is difficult. Again, washing thoroughly will help. Locally grown produce will also have lower pesticide levels.

5. Always buy organic potatoes, if you eat the skins, as these are available and cheap.

6. Many other foods like meats and dairy produce have low pesticide levels so organic are unnecessary but trim off excess fat.

7. It is most important to buy organic and wholemeal bread, cereals, cereal bars, porridge and flour.

NOTE: Many of the above organic items are not regularly available or are too expensive at UK supermarkets in which case concentrate on buying **organic potatoes, bread, cereals (and cereal products) and porridge** most of which are usually present on the shelves.

CHAPTER 5

IS OUR FOOD SAFE?

ADDITIVES

Preservatives, Colourants and Sweeteners

If you just want to know the dangerous ones and how to avoid them go to Section 3 (below)

- **Practically all the food we buy contains additives**

- **Do not panic as advice is given below on "how to avoid the most dangerous additives"**

- **It makes sense to reduce the number of chemicals eaten**

IN OUR FOOD

- There are over 300 different food additives approved for use by the European Union (all with E numbers)

- Around 2600 flavourings are in use in Europe

- Numerous vitamins and minerals are added

- Artificial trans fats are used

Figure 1. Representing the factory processing of our food and the robotic addition of additives on the conveyor belt

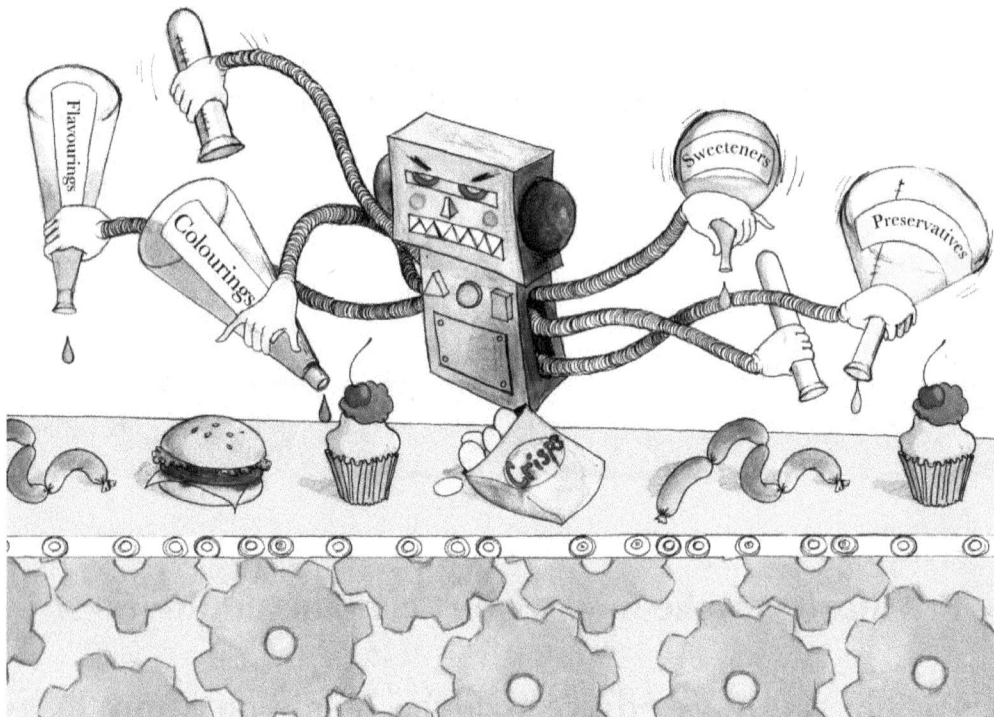

SECTION 1: EXAMPLES OF ADDITIVES PRESENT IN COMMON FOODS AND DRINKS

1. **Muller Light Strawberry, fat-free yoghurt, 200g**
   strawberries (10%)
   beetroot red (E162) and carmine (E120), (colours)
   flavourings (not identified)

aspartame (E951), (sweetener)
citric acid (E330) and sodium citrate (E331), (acidity regulators)
gelatine (E441), (gelling agent)

Total additives = at least 8

2. **SPAR Whole Orange Squash**
    orange from concentrate (10%!)
    potassium sorbate (E202) and sodium metabisulphate (E223), (preservatives)
    beta-carotene (E160a), (colour)
    malic acid (E296) + others (flavourings)
    aspartame (E951) and sodium saccharin (E 954), (sweeteners)
    carboxymethylcellulose (E466), (stabilizer)
    citric acid (E330) and sodium citrate (E331), (acidity regulators)

    Total additives = at least 9

3. **Diet Coke**
    carbonated water
    caramel (E150a), (colour)
    citric acid (E330), (flavouring and preservative)
    caffeine + others? (flavourings)
    phosphoric acid (E338), (flavouring and acidity regulator)
    aspartame (E951) and acesulfame k (E950), (sweeteners)

    Total additives = just water mixed with 5-6 chemicals

WHAT DO YOU THINK OF THE FOLLOWING STATEMENT?

"Soft drinks are an enjoyable source of fluid, which is essential to good health. In combination with a varied diet and regular activity, soft drinks can provide a refreshing and positive contribution to everyday living" from Coca Cola (www.cokeeducation.co.uk).

Comment: Surely, a chemical mixture is not to be preferred to plain water or a 100% pure fruit drink with no additives?

4. **Hot Dog 2 Pack (Snack Express)**

a. roll
calcium propionate (E282). (preservative)
esters of fatty acids (E471, E 472e), (emulsifiers)
vitamin C (E300), (flour treating agent)

b. sausage
sodium nitrite (E250), (preservative)
vitamin C (E300), (antioxidant)
citric acid (flavouring and preservative)
monosodium glutamate (E621), (flavour enhancer)
potassium polymetaphosphate (E452), (stabiliser)
glucono-delta-lactone (E575), (acidity regulator)

c. ketchup
potassium sorbate (E202), (preservative)
flavouring (not identified)

d. mustard
flavouring (not identified)

Total additives = 13 including:

3 preservatives, 1 antioxidant, 4 flavourings, 2 emulsifiers, 1 stabiliser, 1 acidity regulator, 1 flour treating agency plus 3.6 g salt (over half of recommended daily allowance = RDA level).

Remember, many similar and even worse examples can easily be found on any supermarket shelf. For example, a small Nutrigrain Soft Bake Bar has over 16 such additives. **Unfortunately, additives are often associated with the sweets, biscuits, cakes and soft drinks eaten and drunk by our children.**

SECTION 2: TYPES OF ADDITIVES AND THEIR ROLES IN OUR FOOD

Additives approved of by the European Union are labelled on food either by name or have been given an "E" number. In Europe, the "E" numbers indicate that the additives have apparently been tested for safety by the EU (see reference 29 for a full list).

The E numbers of a large number of additives generally fall into the following groups:

- Food colourants are usually E100 to E180.

- Preservatives are mainly E200 to E285.

- Antioxidants are mainly E300 to E321.

- Many thickeners, emulsifiers, stabilisers and gelling agents are included in E400 to E495.

- Many artificial sweeteners are included in E420, E421 and E950-E968.

- There are many other additives with E numbers, such as anti-caking agents and acidity regulators, with numbers going as high as E1500. The numbering scheme misses out many numbers including the 700-800s etc.

1. COLOURANTS (42 approved)

These maintain the natural colour lost in food during processing or storage and also increase the attractiveness of food to the consumer. They are also used to colour artificial "foods" such as sweets or candy and include both natural and synthetic chemical dyes. **Artificially coloured foods are often targeted at children and some sweets, biscuits and desserts may contain multiple colourants**. There is concern that children consume much higher doses of colourants than adults and one study has estimated that they may take in 35-40 different doses of over 12 different colours per day! There are worries (see Section 3 "Safety Concerns", below) about the effects upon children's behaviour of some of the **synthetic azo dyes** commonly used in sweets, soft drinks and ice cream and particularly:

i. Tartrazine (E102)

ii. Quinoline yellow (E104)

iii. Sunset yellow (E110)

iv. Carmoisine or **Azorubine** (E122)

v. Ponceau 4R or **Cochineal Red A** (E124)

vi. Allura Red (E129)

2. PRESERVATIVES (37 approved)

These prevent spoiling of food during transportation and storage. Older preservation techniques include boiling, refrigeration and pickling, as well as the use of salt and sugar. More recently, chemical preservatives have been introduced and are designed to kill bacteria and moulds contaminating food. There are, however, Safety Concerns (see, Section 3, below) in the use of some of these chemicals. These chemicals are designed to increase the shelf-life of food and include:

i. Sulphur dioxide (E220) for dried fruit

ii. Nitrites (E249, 250) and **Nitrates** (E251, 252) with bacon, sausages, ham, corned beef and nearly all cooked meats

iii. Benzoates (E210-213) and **Sorbates** (E200, E201, 202 and 203) are very widely used, especially in soft drinks such as carbonated, squash and still drinks as well as winemaking

3. ANTIOXIDANTS (17 approved)

These include natural antioxidants as well as synthetic antioxidants and are added to food as preservatives to inhibit microbial activity. They also prevent food spoilage caused by exposure to oxygen as seen with the browning of cut potatoes and apples. Two naturally-occurring antioxidants often used are:

i. Vitamin C (ascorbic acid, E300)

ii. Vitamin E (tocopherols, E306)

These vitamin antioxidants are also widely used in foods containing fats or oils to prevent discoloration and odours resulting from contact with oxygen or enzymes which turn fats such as butter rancid (=oxidation). Oxidation of the fats and oils is inhibited by Vitamins C and E that interact with (scavenge) the oxygen. More controversial (see, Section 3 "Safety Concerns", below) is the use of petroleum-based and synthetic antioxidants such as:

iii. Butylated hydroxyanisole (BHA, E320)

iv. Butylated hydroxytoluene (BHT, E321)

4. THICKENERS, EMULSIFIERS, STABILIZERS, ANTI-CAKING AGENTS, ACIDITY REGULATORS, GELLING AGENTS etc (205 approved)

These, for example, thicken soups, maintain mayonnaise in suspension, and prevent lumps forming in salt and flour. Examples are:

i. Pectin (E449) **and Gelatin** (E441) for thickening and stabilizing foods, such as desserts and ice cream allowing them to set and the components to remain in suspension

ii. Lecithin (E322) is an emulsifier and maintains oil, vinegar and water mixed together in suspension in mayonnaise and salad dressings

iii. Calcium silicate (E552) **and silicon dioxide** (E551) are anti-caking agents used to maintain the free flow and prevent lumps forming in powdered food like salt and drinking chocolate

5. ARTIFICIAL SWEETENERS (15 approved)

These are used widely to replace sugar as they contain fewer calories. They are present in so-called "low calorie", "lite" and "low sugar" biscuits, sweets, chewing gum, jams, fizzy and soft drinks, and diet desserts such as yoghurts. The following commonly used, so-called "intense sweeteners" are even sweeter than sugar itself and used at very low concentrations:

i. Acesulfame-K (E950)

ii. Aspartame (E951)

iii. Cyclamate or Cyclamic Acid (E952)

iv. Saccharin (E954)

v. Sucralose (E955)

There has been widespread debate over the safety of these intense sweeteners, especially for children, as they are widely used as sugar substitutes in drinks such as "Coca-Cola Zero", "Fanta", "Sprite", "Dr Pepper" and "Lilt" as well as other soft drinks and squashes (see, Section 3, "Safety Concerns", below).

Other artificial sweeteners include:

vi. Sorbitol (E420)

vii. Mannitol (E421)

These are about 60% as sweet as sugar, and used in similar amounts to sugar, but contain fewer calories and are particularly useful for dieters and for sweetening foods for diabetics.

6. FLAVOUR ENHANCERS AND FLAVOURINGS

i. Flavour enhancers are added to food and drinks to bring out their natural taste. Simple examples used commonly are salt and vinegar. Another example is **monosodium glutamate** (MSG, E621) which is widely used in Chinese food, barbecue sauces, snack foods, frozen dinners and stock cubes.

ii. Flavourings are added to a wide range of foods to give a particular taste or smell. Flavourings can be natural or artificial and at present there are 2600 flavourings in use in the European Union. These additives have not been given E numbers. The European Food Safety Authority (**www.efsa.europa.eu**) intends to evaluate the safety of all flavourings and produce a list authorized for use in the EU. Unfortunately, **food labels often indicate the use of flavourings but fail to name them** so that tighter controls are required (see, Section 3, "Safety Concerns" below, for both MSG and flavourings).

7. NUTRITIONAL ADDITIVES

These include vitamins A, B, C and D, as well as iron, calcium and zinc which are added to fortify some bread, cereals, flour, milk and margarine. Many foods are fortified in the UK and readers should check the labels, particularly of children's sugary cereals and drinks, and realize that these foods are often fortified because of their poor nutritional value.

TRANS FATS (HYDROGENATED FATS)

These are artificially made by passing hydrogen through liquid vegetable oils until they solidify. By this method, margarines were developed as alternative spreads to butter. The food industry readily adopted them as they are cheap padding agents for more expensive foods and also improve both the texture and shelf-life of food.

- However, **trans fats in many studies have been shown to be linked to the development of coronary heart disease** (see reference 30)

- Trans fats are found in fast (junk) food such as chicken nuggets, french fries, as well as in fritters, potato crisps, pizza, ice-cream, puddings, pies, cakes and cake mixes, biscuits, doughnuts, gravy and sauce mixes, confectionery and many other processed foods, including some children's high-sugar breakfast cereals. They are also present in restaurant food and can be formed too by repeatedly re-heating cooking oil

SECTION 3: SAFETY CONCERNS

The European Food Safety Authority (EFSA) is responsible for the safety evaluation of additives for the EU while in the UK the Food Standards Agency (FSA) monitors the safety and use of food additives. The Food and Drug Administration (FDA) controls the use of food additives in the USA.

Despite the fact that food additives in Europe have been given "E" numbers, indicating that they have apparently been tested for safety and approved by the EU, **frequent concerns have arisen as to the wisdom of adding so many chemicals to our food.**

Many people are concerned about food additives and are probably not reassured by Government Agencies. Who can ever forget the BSE crisis and the graphic assurances by the minister in charge that our beef was safe?

On the other hand, it is necessary to maintain a balanced view since many food additives are naturally-occurring substances and harmless, such as the colourants, paprika (E160c), lycopene (E160d) and curcumin (E100). Some food additives, such as salt (within the 6gm limit per day) and vinegar (contains acetic acid, E260), have even been used for hundreds of years with no adverse effects reported.

There is no doubt that additional careful testing of food additives is required as indicated by recent findings that a cocktail of artificial colourants together with the preservative, sodium benzoate, increases hyperactivity in children (McCann and colleagues, The Lancet, Vol. 370, pages 1560 - 1567, 2007, reference 31). Previously, in the 1980s, it had been reported that there was no evidence that such colourants or food additives caused hyperactivity in children.

MAIN FOOD ADDITIVES OF CONCERN

1. COLOURANTS E100-180 may trigger hives, urticaria, asthma and generalized allergic reactions. Of particular concern are the so-called **"azo dyes"** which are widely used in hundreds of food products and medicines. Azo dyes are **synthetic colourants** extracted from crude oil but in the body some:

- **May be cancer-forming**

- **Are also suspected of triggering allergies and behaviour/learning problems in children such as attention deficit hyperactivity disorder (ADHD)**

- **As well as allergies such as asthma, itching, rhinitis and stomach upsets occur especially in those with aspirin sensitivity/allergy**

Following the McCann and colleagues study published in The Lancet, 2007 (see, above = reference 31), the Foods Standard Agency called for a voluntary ban by the end of 2009 on the first 6 dyes in the list in Table 1 (below). The EU also requires food containing these dyes to be labelled "may have an adverse effect on activity and attention of children".

Major shops in the UK, including Tesco, Marks and Spencer, Iceland, Co-op and Asda, either do not use these six colourants or have removed them from their OWN BRAND products.

Food manufacturers also producing foods free of these six colourants include Unilever, Nestle, Cadbury, Trebor Bassett, Heinz (Heinz, Weight Watchers, HP, and Lea & Perrins), Worldfoods, Vimto Soft Drinks (Sunkist, Panda and Vimto) as well as McDonald's OWN BRAND food and drinks.

THERE ARE 16 COLORANTS OF CONCERN [*]:

i. **Tartrazine** (E102)

ii. **Quinoline Yellow** (E104)

iii. **Sunset Yellow** also called **Orange Yellow S** (E110)

iv. **Carmoisine** also called **Azorubine** (E122)

v. **Ponceau 4R** also called **Cochineal Red A** (E124)

vi. **Allura Red** (E129)

vii. **Amaranth** (E123)

viii. **Erythrosine** (E127)

ix. **Red 2G** (E128)

x. **Patent Blue V** (E131)

xi. **Indigo Carmine** (E132)

xii. **Brilliant Blue FCF** (E133)

xiii. **Ammonia Caramel** (150c)

xiv. **Brilliant Black BN** also called **Black PN** (E151)

xv. **Brown FK** (E154)

xvi. **Brown HT or Chocolate Brown HT** (E155)

* For a list of permitted food colourants in the EU see reference 32

Figure 2. Showing a bowl of sweets and the E numbers of colourants used as additives

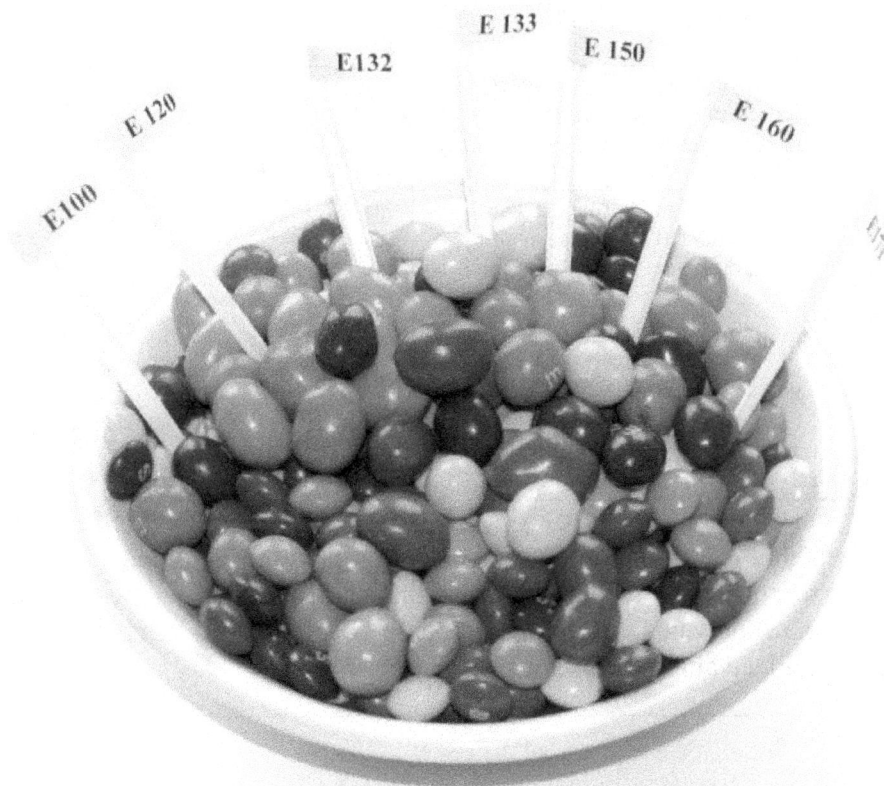

Table 1.   COLOURANT ADDITIVES CAUSING SAFETY CONCERNS

Colourant Name	Present in which foods	Safety Concerns and Possible Health Effects
The first 6 colourants are the azo dyes included in the McCann and colleagues (2007) research[1] and linked to hyperactivity in children. Remove these from the diet.		
i. Tartrazine (E102)	Yellow, in soft drinks, sweets, ices, jams, cereals, cake mixes, mustard, yoghurts, some package soups, and tinned foods	Linked to hyperactivity and ADHD[2] in children, as well as allergies associated with itching, rhinitis, migraine, asthma etc. Banned in Austria, Germany and Norway
ii. Quinoline Yellow (E104)	Soft drinks, cough sweets, ices, scotch eggs, chewing gum, and smoked haddock. Also, in lipstick and children's medicines	Linked to hyperactivity and ADHD[2] in children, as well as allergies, such as dermatitis. May damage genes and cause cancer. Banned in Australia, Japan, Norway and USA
iii. Sunset Yellow (E110)	Soft drinks, sweets, ices, jellies, trifle, apricot jam, marzipan, lemon curd, Swiss roll, hot chocolate and packet soups. Also, breadcrumbs, cheese sauce, canned fish, and children's medicines	Linked to hyperactivity and ADHD[2] in children and allergic reactions and can result in stomach upsets, nettle rash etc. Sometimes contaminated with Sudan I, a banned cancer forming azo dye. Banned in Canada, Japan, Scandinavia and USA
iv. Carmoisine (Azorubine) (E122)	Red dye in soft drinks, sweets, jellies, marzipan, yoghurt, cheesecakes and children's medicines	Linked to hyperactivity and ADHD[2] in children and allergic reactions such as skin rash in asthmatics. Banned in Japan, Norway, Sweden and USA
v. Ponceau 4R (E124)= Cochineal Red A	Red dye in some drinks, sweets, cakes, dessert toppings, salami, salad dressings, cheesecakes and trifles	Linked to hyperactivity and ADHD[2] in children and can produce bad reactions in asthmatics. Regarded as cancer-forming in animals. Banned in Finland Norway and USA
vi. Allura Red (E129)	In soft drinks, sweets, biscuits, cereals, condiments and medicines	Linked to hyperactivity and ADHD[2] in children, and may produce bad reactions in people allergic to aspirin. Linked with cancer in mice. Banned in Austria, Belgium, France, Germany, Scandinavia and Switzerland
The following colourants include azo dyes, but were not tested in the McCann and colleagues research[1]. They may also cause behavioural/learning problems in children, as well as allergic reactions and even cancer in adults but proof is sometimes incomplete. All food colourants must now be labelled. Colorants E100 - E180 may trigger hives, urticaria, asthma and generalized allergic reactions.		

vii. Amaranth (E123)	Purple-red azo dye in some blackcurrant and red soft and alcoholic drinks, ice creams, jams, jellies, tinned fruit, trifle, cake mixes, prawns, gravy granules, soups and medicines	Linked to allergies, asthma, eczema and hyperactivity in children. Numerous studies link it to cancer in laboratory animals, birth defects, stillbirths, sterility and early foetal death. Banned in Austria, Norway, Russia, United States, and with restricted use in France and Italy (caviar only)
viii. Erythrosine (E127)	Pink-red, non-azo, synthetic, coal tar dye in sweets, biscuits, cakes, glace cherries, strawberries and rhubarb, packet desserts, spreads and patés, processed cooked meat	Potentially causing thyroid problems and reduces sperm count in animals, potential factor in breast cancer. Recommended for banning in USA
ix. Red 2G (E128)	Azo dye found in some breakfast sausages and burgers	Potentially cancer-forming. The EFSA[3] banned it's use in 2007 including in UK. Already banned in many countries such as Norway and USA
x. Patent Blue V (E 131)	A non-azo, synthetic, coal tar dye not widely used in foods but in sweets, occasional soft drink and scotch eggs. Also, in plaque disclosing tablets and injected to trace blood vessels	Linked to allergies, nettle rash, itching, low blood pressure and occasional serious allergic shock. Banned in Australia, Japan, Norway, New Zealand USA
xi. Indigo Carmine (E132)	Blue, non-azo, synthetic dye, derived from coal tar. Found in sweets, ice cream, baked goods, confectionary, biscuits, as well as tablets and capsules	In people such as asthmatics, may cause nausea, vomiting, high blood pressure, skin rashes, breathing problems and other allergic reactions. Banned in Norway
xii. Brilliant Blue FCF (E133)	Non-azo, synthetic dye from coal tar. Often found in sweets, ice cream, dairy products, drinks, tinned peas, cosmetics and soaps	Hyperactive Children's Support Group (HACSG)[4] recommends elimination from children's diets. Cancer induction unproven? EU approved. Banned previously in Austria, Belgium, France, Germany Norway, Sweden and Switzerland
xiii. Ammonia Caramel (E150c)	Non-azo dye widely used in chocolates, ice cream, soft drinks, beer, wine, whiskey bakery goods, pickles, sauces, snacks	Possible allergen. Reports of adverse effects on hyperactivity, and toxicity to stomach, liver, reproduction and blood need confirmation
xiv. Brilliant Black BN (E151)	Azo dye found in soft drinks, flavored milk, sweets, ice cream, blackcurrant cake mixes, food decorations, desserts, jellies, red fruit jams, mustard, brown sauces, fish paste etc	HACSG[4] recommends elimination from children's diets. May damage genes and cause cancer. Banned in Australia, much of Western Europe and USA
xv. Brown FK (E154)	Azo dye found in smoked fish, cooked meat and crisps	Similar concerns to Brilliant Blue (E133), including hyperactivity and ADHD
xvi. Brown HT (E155)	An azo dye found mainly in chocolate flavour cakes.	Similar concerns to Brilliant Blue (E133), including hyperactivity and ADHD[2]

1. McCann and colleagues, The Lancet, Vol. 370, pages 1560 - 1567, 2007, reference 31
2. ADHD =attention deficit hyperactivity disorder

3. EFSA is the European Food Safety Authority **(www.efsa.europa.eu)**
4. HACSG is the Hyperactive Children's Support Group **(www.hacsg.org.uk)**

BOTTOM LINE ON FOOD COLOURANTS

BE PARTICULARLY CONCERNED FOR POSSIBLE EFFECTS ON:

- Children - may induce allergies and behavioural effects

- Adults - may induce or aggravate allergies

Note also:

- That many cosmetics and some children's medicines contain azo dyes (see reference 33)

- Manufacturers are removing these colourants from many sweets and medicines although the latter still contain sulphite preservatives (see, Table 2, below)

2/3. PRESERVATIVES AND ANTIOXIDANTS

TABLE 2. PRESERVATIVE AND ANTIOXIDANT ADDITIVES CAUSING SAFETY CONCERNS

Preservative Name	Present in which Foods	Safety Concerns and Possible Health Effects
i. **Sorbates E200-203** Sorbic acid (E200) Sodium sorbate (E201) Potassium sorbate (E202) Calcium sorbate (E203)	Widely used anti - microbial agents, found in soft drinks, sweets, wine, cakes, pies, pickles, salad dressings, sauces, dairy products (not milk drinks), dry fruits, fish, beauty /health products etc	**Generally recognized as safe by JECFA [1], FDA [2] and the FSA [3].** However, sorbic acid has been shown to interact with nitrite preservative to form low levels of cancer–forming agents but none of these have been shown to transform cells [4]. Sorbic acid may cause skin irritation.
ii. **Benzoates E210-214** Benzoic acid (E210) Sodium benzoate (E211) Potassium benzoate (E212) Calcium benzoate (E213) Ethyl 4-hydroxybenzoate (E214)	Widely used anti-microbial agents, found in soft drinks, sweets, jellies, jams, cakes, pickles, salad dressings, sauces, crisps, child medicines, beauty and health products etc	**Whether sodium benzoate (E211) is safe is controversial.** E211 was mixed with azo dyes in the McCann et al., (2007) study [5] on azo dyes linked to hyperactivity in children. The FSA [3] banned these dyes but not E211. Benzoates may aggravate asthma and allergies and HACSG [6] suggests avoidance. E211 can interact with vitamin C in soft drinks to form the cancer–forming compound, benzene. There is evidence for damage to DNA in cells [7]. Parents should prevent children from drinking too many soft drinks with E211 and azo dyes.
iii. **Sulphites E220-228** Sulphur dioxide (E220) Sodium sulphite (E221) Sodium bisulphite (E222) Sodium metabisulphite (E223) Potassium metabisulphite (E224) Calcium sulphite (E226) Calcium bisulphite (E227) Potassium bisulphite (E228)	Anti-microbial agents, used in soft drinks and fruit juices, jams, sausages, beer, wine, yoghurt, potato products, frozen shellfish, pickles, balsamic vinegar and **often in dried fruits**. In beer and wine but may not be labelled. Also in medicines (including children's), cosmetics, beauty and hair care products.	**Much concern over safety of sulphites. In USA FDA [2] prohibits use on fresh fruit and vegetables** including peeled potatoes to stop browning. Can provoke sneezing, breathing problems etc in asthmatics and even severe shock. Sulphites have been included among the top 10 substances causing allergies. Some antihistamines medicines may contain sodium bisulphite! Some sulphites also destroy vitamin B1 (thiamin). In UK sulphite levels in food above 10mg per kg or litre should be labelled.

iv. **Nitrites and Nitrates (E249-252)** Potassium nitrite (E249) Sodium nitrite (E250) Sodium nitrate (E 251) Potassium nitrate (E 252)	Antibacterial agents, colour and flavour stabilizers used in cured and smoked meats such as ham, bacon, tongue, hot dogs, corned beef, sausages, salami, luncheon meat, as well as fish. Beware burnt or charred red meat such as crispy fried bacon. Also, present in cosmetics.	**Much media concern for safety of nitrites and nitrates used in cured meats as they can be converted in the body into cancer-forming nitrosamines.** However, it has been estimated that only about 5% of your daily intake of nitrosamines comes from cured meat with most derived from vegetables and drinking water (from nitrates used as fertilizers), cigarette smoke, cars etc. Even so, the EFSA[8] and FSA[3] have reduced the levels of potassium and sodium nitrates allowed in meat products. Sodium nitrite may induce hyperactivity and HACSG [6] suggests avoidance. Vitamin C and E may block cancer-forming nitrosamines[9].
v. **Butylated hydroxyanisole (BHA) (E 320)**	Antioxidant preservative, in UK mainly used in butter, margarine, lard and vegetable oils to prevent them becoming rancid or bad. Also in sweets, cereals, chewing gum, potato chips, meats, nuts, lipstick and eye shadow	**Suspected as a cancer-inducing agent although evidence inconclusive.** May interact in stomach with nitrites to produce cancer-forming compounds. Also, limited evidence of association with allergic or intolerance responses such as asthma and rhinitis. Now being replaced by natural antioxidants such as vitamins E and C. Should not be present in infants' food. Banned in Japan and by McDonalds in USA.
vi. **Butylated hydroxytoluene (BHT) (E 321)**	See E320, above	See E320, above

1. JECFA is World Health Organisation (WHO) Expert Committee on Food Additives
2. FDA is US Food and Drug Administration (**www.cfsan.fda.gov/~dms/fdsweet.html**)
3. FSA is Food Standards Agency, UK (**www.food.gov.uk**)
4. See reference 34
5. See reference 31
6. HACSG is the Hyperactive Children's Support Group (**www.hacsg.org.uk**)
7. See reference 35
8. EFSA is the European Food Safety Authority (**www.efsa.europa.eu**)
9. See reference 36

BOTTOM LINE ON CHEMICAL FOOD PRESERVATIVES AND ANTIOXIDANTS

- Sorbates are recognised as the safest group of preservatives.

- Children are particularly vulnerable to the effects of preservatives due to excessive intakes in soft drinks and sweets.

- More "natural" preservatives are now being researched and introduced slowly.

- Levels of some chemical preservatives in food are being reduced by FSA and EFSA legislation.

- Cured meats labelled "naturally cured" or "no added nitrite" may contain nitrite from plant material high in nitrates and used for curing.

- NB: Many cosmetics, beauty and hair products may also contain chemical preservatives.

4. ARTIFICIAL SWEETENERS. The most widely used and those causing safety concerns are included in Table 3, below.

Table 3.   ARTIFICIAL SWEETENERS CAUSING SAFETY CONCERNS

Sweetener Name	Present in which Foods	Safety Concerns and Possible Health Effects
i. Acesulphame K (E950)	Marketed as "Sunette", "Ace K" and "Sweet One". Used widely in soft drinks such as Diet Coke and alcoholic drinks. Also in sweets, ice cream, desserts, jams, dairy products, baked goods, chewing gum, dressings, body builders' protein drinks, toothpaste, mouthwash, cosmetics, medicines	Acesulphame has been widely tested and is generally recognized as safe by JECFA[1], FDA[2] and the FSA[3]. It is approved for use in many countries. There have, however, been adverse reports suggesting cancer-forming properties[4] and suggestions of the need for additional testing[5]. Furthermore, acesulphame, like all artificial sweeteners, may affect the blood sugar and increase food cravings? Banned from young children's products

ii. **Aspartame** **(E951)**	Marketed as "Equal", "Canderel", and "NutraSweet". Found in about 6000 foods Worldwide such as soft drinks, sweets, desserts, chewing gum, dairy products, cakes, biscuits, jams, vitamin and mineral pills, weight-control products, as a substitute for sugar in hot drinks, and in medicines	**Aspartame has been recognized as safe by FDA[2], FSA[3] and EFSA[6] and has been in use over 25 years.** Despite numerous studies confirming it's safety, reports of neurological and behavioural problems have appeared, often after very high doses. Public concern persists especially after induction of tumours in rats[7]. People with phenylketonuria disease should avoid aspartame as it contains phenylalanine which they cannot break down. In the UK, Asda is removing aspartame from the "Good for You" range of foods. Children's drinks containing aspartame should be avoided /diluted. Banned in Philippines
iii. **Cyclamate** **(Cyclamic acid)** **(E952)**	Marketed as "Sucaryl" (which is combined with 1 part saccharin to 10 parts cyclamate). Not used in UK until 1995 and found mainly in soft drinks and squashes. Other foods sold containing cyclamates may be imported and include cakes, biscuits, chocolate, jams, cereals, sugar-free chewing gum and breath-freshening sweets, as well as pharmaceuticals	**Cyclamates approved for use by WHO[1] and EFSA[6] but banned in USA since 1970** due to report of bladder cancer in rats fed a blend of cyclamate/saccharin (10 parts:1 part), and of damage to testes in mice fed cyclamate. In contrast, over 75 recent studies failed to show any toxicity to humans and approved for use in over 50 countries. However, safety concerns persist, particularly for 1½-4½ yr children drinking more than 3 beakers (180 ml each) of diluted squashes/soft drinks per day, as the ADI (acceptable daily intake) of cyclamate is then exceeded. The FSA[3] advises increasing dilution of squash/soft drinks for young children to reduce cyclamate intake
iv. **Saccharin** **(E954)**	Marketed as "Sweet'N Low," "SweetTwin" and "Necta Sweet" (in USA). Used as table top sweetener and found in drinks, sweets, jams, salad dressings, chewing gum, toothpaste, vitamins and medicines	**Saccharin safety is approved by JECFA[1] and EFSA[6] and in use in over 90 countries but controversial** due to reports of formation of bladder cancer in rats fed high doses of saccharin throughout their lives. Derived from coal tar. Recent research, however, has mainly shown that saccharin is safe for humans due to their different physiology to rats. Generally, evidence "does not link saccharin and human bladder cancer" at the present time. Banned in Canada
v. **Sucralose** **(E955)**	Marketed as "Splenda". Used widely as table top sweetener and found in soft drinks, ice cream, fruit juices, milk products, puddings, baked goods, sweets, coffee, tea, canned fruit, jam, breakfast snack bars, sauces and chewing gum	**Sucralose is generally regarded as safe and approved by JECFA[1], FDA[2], and EFSA[6] It is a recently developed sweetener** (in use in last 10-15 years). In use in over 40 counties including USA and Europe, Brazil, China, Japan, Australia. Safety concluded by FDA[2] from over 110 studies of animals and humans. Even so there appears to be a lack of long-term studies in humans and this coupled with the chlorine content of sucralose has raised safety concerns. The presence of chlorine or chloride in a substance does not indicate toxicity as common salt contains chloride!

vi. Other sweeteners eg. "Neotame"(E961), and "Stevia"	Other sweeteners are being introduced that are artificial, such as Neotame (E961), or natural, such as Stevia (no E number)	Neotame is approved by the FDA[2] and JECFA[1] and has no safety concerns for the EFSA[6]. Neotame is made from aspartame (see above) so similar safety concerns apply. Stevia is naturally derived from a plant but even so is not approved in USA or Europe. NOTE: because a substance is natural does not guarantee its safety

1. JECFA is World Health Organisation (WHO) Expert Committee on Food Additives
2. FDA is US Food and Drug Administration (**www.cfsan.fda.gov/~dms/fdsweet.html**)
3. FSA is Food Standards Agency, UK (**www.food.gov.uk**)
4. See reference 37
5. **http://www.cspinet.org/reports/asekquot.html**
6. EFSA is the European Food Safety Authority (**www.efsa.europa.eu**)
7. See reference 38

BOTTOM LINE ON ARTIFICIAL SWEETENERS:

- A huge range of foods and drinks contain artificial sweeteners so they are difficult to avoid.

- Many foods containing sweeteners are highly processed and of low nutritional value i.e. junk foods such as soft drinks, cakes and sweets.

- Of concern is the fact that children and teenagers consume particularly high levels of artificially sweetened junk foods and therefore ingest high doses of these additives.

- Food, drink and medicines containing artificial sweeteners are not recommended for babies (and actually banned in baby foods) and very young children (less than 3 yr) as they have rapidly developing bodies which may be particularly vulnerable to any bad effects.

- Many artificial sweeteners are often used in combinations such as **"Sweet'N Low",** which is a mixture of acesulfame and aspartame, and widely used in coffee shops.

- All ADIs (acceptable daily intakes) are calculated for each additive when used alone but evidence indicates that mixtures of additives, such as sweeteners, may be more toxic (see Chapter 6 "The Cocktail Effect").

- Most "diet", "light" or "zero" products contain artificial sweeteners. The public is being exposed to a high-powered advertising campaign trying to promote these chemical mixes to gullible children and adults.

5. FLAVOUR ENHANCERS AND FLAVOURINGS. As mentioned above (see page 98), **2600 flavourings** are used in foods and drinks in the European Union but have not been given E numbers since the majority have **not been tested for safety**. Many food labels mention the addition of flavourings but fail to identify them. The European Food Safety Authority (**www.efsa.europa.eu)** intends to rectify this by evaluating the safety of all flavourings. Flavour enhancers intensify and enhance flavours of food without necessarily having a taste of their own. One such flavour enhancer is Monosodium Glutamate (MSG) or 'Hydrolyzed Vegetable Protein,' as it is sometimes labelled on food. MSG is widely used, has received much attention and has also been given an E number, E621.

Monosodium glutamate (E621)

Foods present in: Processed food including sausages, pies, sauces, soups, crisps, stock cubes, noodles, Chinese food, tin foods, fast foods, ready meals and some cheeses.

Safety concerns and possible health effects: MSG has been regarded as safe by JECFA[1], FDA[2] and EFSA[3] when consumed at an approximate average daily intake of up to 10g/day. In addition, no mutagenicity (cancer potential) has been reported. However, many consumers have reported adverse side effects including the "Chinese Restaurant Syndrome" characterized by headache, throbbing of the head, dizziness, nausea, sweating, flushing, wheezing, burning or tingling sensations over parts of the body, as well as chest pain, and back pain. Many of the side effects of MSG are regarded as unproven.

There is, however, some evidence of adverse effects of MSG. For example, it has recently been shown that MSG enhances liver damage induced by trans fatty acids[4] (see Chapter 3, Table 1) and may be linked to obesity by enhancing food intake[5]. Also, it has been shown that MSG can induce oxidative stress which could potentially damage organs such as testes as well as DNA, although levels of MSG given to animals were very high. Finally, MSG is chemically similar to glutamate, one of the brains messenger molecules. It may well be able to cross into the developing brains of newborns and young children and possibly cause damage. The Co-op supermarket has banned MSG from its own label foods and many food producers no longer add MSG to their baby foods.

1. JECFA is World Health Organisation (WHO) Expert Committee on Food Additives
2. FDA is US Food and Drug Administration (**www.cfsan.fda.gov/~dms/fdsweet.html**)
3. EFSA is the European Food Safety Authority (**www.efsa.europa.eu**)
4. See reference 39
5. See reference 40

6. TRANS FATS (HYDROGENATED FATS). See Chapter 3 for details of health concerns.

SUMMARY AND HOW TO REDUCE ADDITIVES IN YOUR DIET

- Thousands of foods and drinks contain additives so it is virtually impossible to entirely eliminate all of these from your diet.

- Many of these additives are not essential but purely added to improve colour or taste of food lost during processing.

- Because an additive has been deemed "safe" does not mean that it is good for you. Many **highly processed foods** with lots of colourants, flavourings and sweeteners contain very few ingredients of any value to the body.

- Understand that safe levels of additives (the ADI or <u>a</u>cceptable <u>d</u>aily <u>i</u>ntakes) are calculated for each additive when used **on its own** but mixtures of additives, found in many products, may interact and **greatly magnify their toxicity/side effects** (see Chapter 6, "The Cocktail Effect").

- Reduce or avoid food additives especially if you or your family have young children or have other members suffering from allergies (see: <u>www.hacsg.org.uk</u> for advice) or are pregnant.

- Unborn babies and young children with rapidly developing bodies will be **particularly vulnerable** to any harmful effects of additives.

- Check medicines and vitamins for young children as these may contain additives banned from foods.

- Avoid sulphite (E220-228) and benzoate (E21-214) preservatives as well as artificial colourants (Table 1, above) as this may help reduce allergic responses.

- Dilute squash/soft drinks for young (less than 4.5 yr) children to reduce cyclamate sweetener intake.

- For details of what additives are present in children's foods consult <u>www.netmums.com/food/Action_on_Additives.992</u> and <u>www.foodcomm.org.uk/parentsjury/add_2.htm</u>

The easiest way of avoiding additives is to drink water, buy locally grown fresh fruit and vegetables, and read food labels to find out what chemical additives are present in your food. A limited number of organic foods are also recommended (see Chapter 4)

- Organic food is much safer with only 36 additives allowed as opposed to 100s or even 1000s (if you include flavourings) in non-organic food.

- **The good news is that** Sainsbury, Marks and Spencer, Tesco and Asda are removing many additives from their **own brand products**. Britvic is removing sodium benzoate out of drinks aimed at children such as some of the Robinson's range.

- However, these supermarkets **still import foreign foods with dangerous additives**. For example, Sainsbury's own brand pasta is free of trans fats and yet they still sell Italian pasta with trans fats labelled-WHY?

- Beware the terms "healthy" and "natural" found on labels. To check the flavourings in a drink/food look at the label and if it contains real fruit extract then it is natural but if it contains a list of chemicals then it is artificially flavoured.

- Finally, although controversial, products with artificial sweeteners might encourage you to eat more/consume more calories, and put on weight.

CHAPTER 6

THE COCKTAIL EFFECT

OH NO, NOT MORE CHEMICALS!

What is the Total Chemical Load of the Body from ALL SOURCES?

How to Reduce your Body Burden of Chemicals

All Parents Should Read This Chapter Since Babies And Children Are Potentially More Vulnerable Than Adults to Toxic Chemicals

If you just want to know how to avoid the most harmful chemicals present in the environment and how to reduce your "Body Burden" of chemicals then just read Section 5, pages 131-136, below

We have already seen in Chapter 4 on "Pesticides" and Chapter 5 on "Additives" that our bodies are exposed to a large number of chemicals added artificially to our food and drink. In the present Chapter, we reveal additional, potentially toxic chemicals, to which we are exposed to daily from numerous other sources including cosmetics and furnishings.

115

Figure 1. Shows the origin of the many chemicals that we are exposed to and which form a cocktail in the body

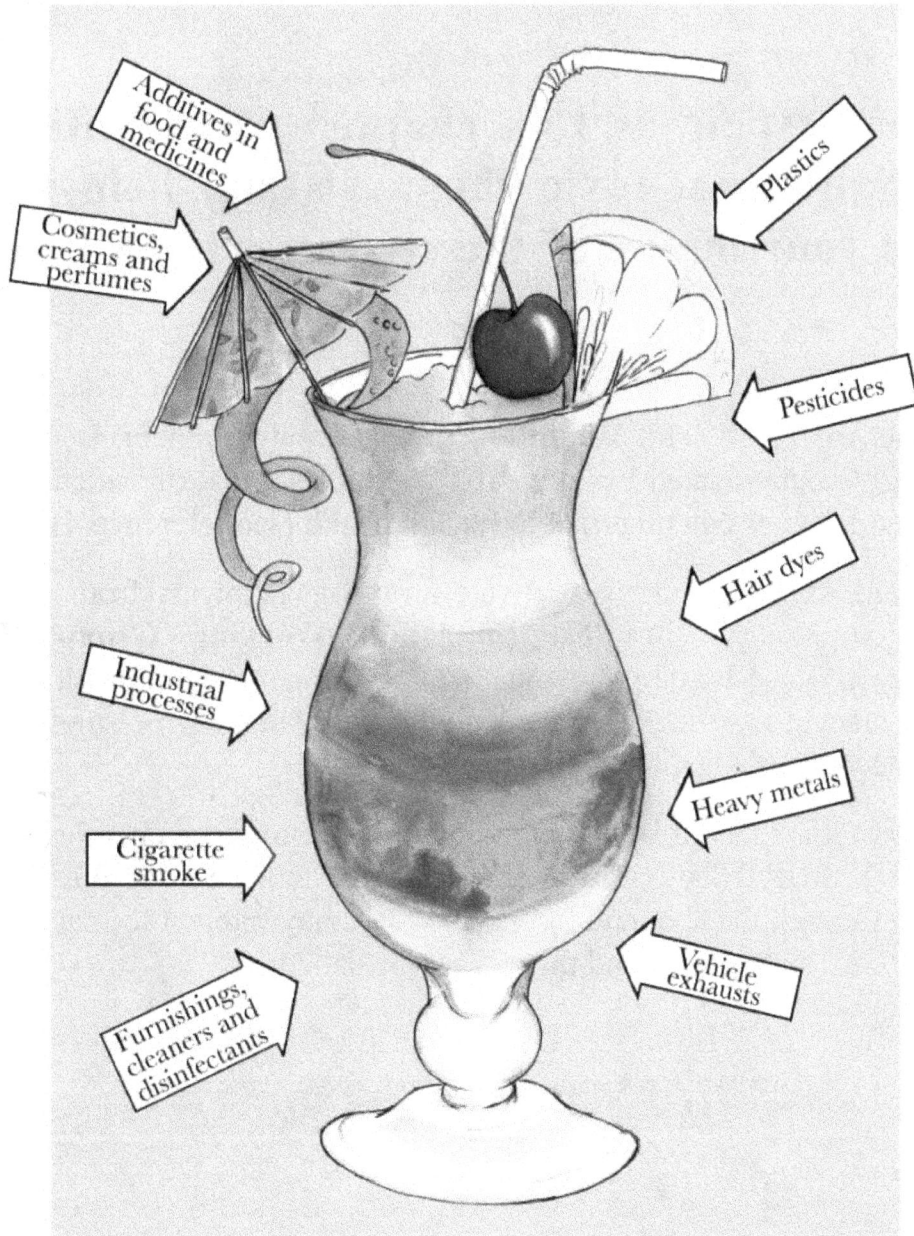

THERE IS NO ESCAPE FROM THESE CHEMICALS

Except to go and live in a deep cave with no modern appliances or furnishings, processed food, drink or consumer products.

In addition, few people have the time or know-how to read and understand minute labels on food, drink, cosmetics etc in order to avoid the most toxic chemicals.

Do not despair as this chapter will identify the potentially most toxic chemicals and help you to reduce your intake of these (see Sections 1 and 5, below).

According to the **World Wildlife Fund** our environment is becoming increasingly contaminated by industrial chemicals, most of which have not been tested for their potential risk to human health (see reference 41).

In addition, we are exposed to a vast array of chemicals from consumer goods. For example, an **Environmental Working Group (EWG)** (<u>www.ewg.org/reports</u>) study showed that "89 percent of 10,500 ingredients used in personal care products have not been evaluated for safety by any publicly accountable institution."

The end result is that our bodies contain a mixture of these chemicals called, the **"BODY BURDEN"**. These chemicals are taken up via our food and drink and through the skin and lungs, and they may interact to magnify their harmful effect on the body and this process is called

"THE COCKTAIL EFFECT"

It is common sense to reduce the numbers of chemicals taken in, as **nobody** knows their long-term cumulative effect, i.e. **"The Cocktail Effect"**, on our health.

A major problem is that although organisations (such as the Food Standards Agency in the UK) set limits on levels of chemicals, including pesticides and additives, they ONLY usually consider individual chemicals on their own. UNFORTUNATELY, mixtures of additives are found in many products and these may accumulate and interact in the body to greatly magnify their toxicity/side effects (See, Section 3, "Synergistic Effects", below).

- **This Chapter deals with:**

1. Sources of chemicals that we are exposed to and which are potentially most toxic

2. The "Body Burden" of these chemicals and which are most commonly found in the tissues of the body

3. Evidence for a synergistic (i.e. interactive) effect of these chemicals

4. Possible harmful effects of the "Body Burden" of chemicals and their link to disease

5. Avoidance/reduction of "Body Burden" of chemicals and strategies for detoxification (detox)

SECTION 1: SOURCES OF CHEMICALS TAKEN INTO THE BODY

The following Table 1 identifies the sources and chemicals of some concern. For additional details, the reader should consult the websites for the **Environmental Working Group (EWG)** (see reference 42), and also for the **World Wildlife Fund** (see reference 41).

Table 1.   SOURCES OF ARTIFICIAL CHEMICALS OF PARTICULAR SAFETY CONCERNS INCLUDED IN "THE COCKTAIL EFFECT"

Source of Chemical	Name of Chemical	Safety Concerns and Possible Health Effects
i. Pesticides In food and drink	**Persistent Organic Pollutants (POPs)**. Include DDT, HCH and aldrin	POPs may cause breast and other cancers, suppress the immune system, disturb hormonal functions and fertility, and pollute human breast milk with short and long-term consequences (see Chapter 4). Not all POPs are pesticides eg. PCBs and dioxins (see xi. and xii., below).
ii. Additives In food, drink and medicines	**Colourants, preservatives, sweeteners** etc. Includes azo dyes, benzoates, sulphites, aspartame	Some **additives** may be involved in cancer formation, behavioural/learning problems in children, as well as the aggravation of allergies and hypersensitivity, and the induction of organ damage through oxidative stress and weight gain (see Chapter 5).
iii. Some cosmetics and makeup, lipstick, moisterizers, suncreams, deodorants, hairsprays, shampoos, perfumes, shaving cream and even in toddlers toothpaste contain mixtures of potentially toxic chemicals	**Parabens** (methyl-,ethyl-, propyl- and butyl- parabens)	**Parabens** are preservatives and have also been approved for use in food and medicines (= E214-219) as well as cosmetics for many years (see reference 43). Parabens are present in human breast cancer tissue. They can mimic the female sex hormone, oestrogen, which has been linked to breast cancer as well as the disruption of sperm production in rats (see reference 44). Parabens can also cause rashes and skin allergies. Parabens may accumulate in women with long term use of cosmetics, particularly of under arm deodorants/perfumes. The FDA[1] and cosmetics producers view is that parabens in cosmetics are safe due to the low levels used BUT neither the "long term accumulation effect" nor the "cocktail effect" have been tested in detail.

iv. Some cosmetics and makeup, lipstick, moisterizers, suncreams, deodorants, hairsprays, shampoos, perfumes, shaving creams and even toddlers toothpaste contain mixtures of potentially toxic chemicals	**Polyethylene glycols (PEGs)** Contaminated with ethylene dioxide, 1,4-dioxane and polycyclic aromatic hydrocarbons (PAH)	**PEGs** keep the ingredients of the cosmetic mixed and help spreading over the skin. Generally, PEGs are regarded as safe although safety tests are incomplete (see reference 45). The main problem is with the contaminants in PEGs. They may contain various harmful impurities including: **Ethylene oxide** which increases the incidences of uterine and breast cancers and of leukemia and brain cancer. **1, 4-dioxane** which according to the US EPA[2] is a "probable human carcinogen" and also causes irritation to the eyes, nose, throat, lungs and skin as well as liver and kidney damage. **Polycyclic aromatic compounds** (PAHs) which are known to increase the risk of breast cancer.
v. Some cosmetics etc, as above, for Parabens and PEGs	**Propylene glycol**	**Popylene glycol** is present in many cosmetics, moisturisers, shampoos, foods and medicines. Regarded as safe in food but may cause allergic reactions in skin (dermatitis) and lungs, irritates the eyes, penetrates the skin and may cause kidney or liver damage.
vi. Common in shampoos, soaps, bubble bath, shower gels, shaving foam, washing up liquid, toothpaste, carpet and floor cleaners, car wash.	**Sodium lauryl sulphate (SLS or SDS)**	**SLS** is a strong detergent/lathering agent and present in over 75% of shampoos and conditioners. It is **highly irritating to the skin in some people** and can trigger dermatitis. The Data Safety Sheet for SLS[3] states "avoid contact with skin and eyes", mutagenic (may cause cancer), may accumulate in the body and cause organ damage, if inhaled get medical attention immediately (!). Also, found in children's products!
vii. Some food, hairsprays, deodorants, nail polish, perfumes, suncreams, table cloths, floor tiles, furnishings, shower curtains, rainwear, dolls, some toys, car upholstery, food packaging, plastic water bottles.	**Phthalates (eg. DBP and DEHP)**	**Phthalates** are added to plastics to make them more flexible and are widely distributed in the environment from factories, leaching from plastic in landfill sites or from burning. They are also released indoors from plastic products. Phthalates have been detected in the blood and urine of most people tested. Phthlataes are hormone disruptors and may increase both the risk of birth defects and reproductive abnormalities as well as breast cancer in women. Exposure to low levels of phthalates may occur from beauty products, by eating food in plastic packages, by breathing dust in rooms with furnishings and by drinking bottled water, all of which may contain phthalates. Some phthalates are banned by European Union from children's soft toys, teething rings and dummies[4]- beware some imports!

viii. In polycarbonate plastics for baby and water bottles, sports equipment, dental fillings, and electronics. Epoxy resins with bisphenol A used to coat the inside of food and drink cans. Bisphenol is also a flame retardant precursor.	**Bisphenol A (BPA)**	**Bisphenol A** is used in a wide range of plastics but most concern is with it's **presence in baby bottles and linings of cans** from which it may leach into food and drink. The FSA[5], the EFSA[6] and the FDA[1] all believe that the amount of BPA to which babies and children are being exposed does "not indicate a safety concern" and is "without appreciable risk". Unfortunately, like phthalates, BPA is another hormone disruptor in animal studies but controversy surrounds the risk of BPA to humans, due to limited studies. The NTP[7] stated that "several studies collectively suggest hormonal effects in humans". With mounting public concern, Canada and several USA States are banning the sale/importation of polycarbonate baby bottles.
ix. Sunscreen, facial moisturisers, lipsticks and lip balm.	**Oxybenzone =** Benzophenone-3	**Oxybenzone** is present in over 40% of sunscreens. It is readily absorbed through the skin and may cause hormone disruption and low birth weight of girls[8]. Much more data required but caution worthwhile.
x. In soft furnishings eg. in foam cushions, mattresses, as well as children's pyjamas, plastics of TVs and computers.	**Flame retardants (eg. polybrominated diphenyl ethers= PBDE)**	**Like pesticides (above), PBDEs are POPs (see i. Pesticides, above)** and enter and persist in the environment and pass up the food chain to be eaten and accumulate in human fat. They then enter human breast milk and pass into the foetus and baby. They are present throughout the environment, in air, water and food, and are impossible to avoid. In mice, they are toxic to the liver, thyroid, and are also neurotoxins and endocrine disruptors. They are banned by the EU but continue to accumulate in landfill sites from old furniture foam and electronics plastic.
xi. Previously, widely used in paints, adhesives, plastics, flame retardants, rubber and electrical goods eg. fluorescent lights. Coolants and lubricants in large electrical equipment – transformers capacitors etc.	**Polychlorinated biphenyls (PCBs).** Include over 100 different compounds.	**PCBs are another group of Persistent Organic Pollutants POPs (see i. Pesticides, above).** Despite the banning of PCBs and other POPS in many countries[9], they are still being found in human tissues. This is due to bioconcentration in food chains, through long-term environmental contamination of soils, water and air by industrial and incineration processes. **As humans are at the top of many food chains we may ingest high levels of these POPs from fish, meat etc.** These residual POPs may cause breast and other cancers, suppress the immune system, disturb hormonal functions and pollute breast milk with unknown short and long-term consequences for babies and infants.

xii. Produced by paper mills, waste incinerators etc, from cigarettes and exhausts. Most dioxins are ingested via full fat dairy produce and meat from animals fed on polluted pastures or feed. Dioxins dissolve in body fat and milk. Also, in poultry, eggs, cereals, fish and fish oils, and unwashed fruit and vegetables.	**Dioxins.** Include a group of about 17 chlorine-containing compounds.	**Dioxins** are another group of Persistent Organic Pollutants POPs (see i. Pesticides, and xi. PCBs, above). They are unintentional products from industry as well as from grass fires, volcanic activity etc. and are found throughout the environment in soils, water and air. They bioaccumulate in food chains into the human diet. The long-term effects, like the PCBs, probably involve the immune system, reproduction and development, including possible hormonal disturbances. Dioxins are also involved in a skin disease called chloracne with widespread pustules over the body. There are strong indications of increased risk of cancers in particular regions of the body and of the cancer-forming potential of dioxins. **The Seveso disaster released high levels of dioxins into adjacent areas and 10 years after the explosion, people were more likely to have cancer**[10]. Like PCBs and other POPs, dioxins are subject to the Stockholm Convention (2001)[9] and countries are obliged to take measures to eliminate and minimise all sources of dioxins.

1. FDA = Food and Drug Administration, USA (**www.fda.gov › Cosmetics**)
2. US EPA = United States Environmental Protection Agency (**www.epa.gov/ttnatw01/hlthef/dioxane.html**)
3. Material Safety Data Sheet for sodium lauryl sulphate (**www.sciencelab.com/xMSDS-Sodium_lauryl_sulfate-9925002**)
4. The Environment Agency (**www.environment-agency.gov.uk/business/39127.aspx**)
5. FSA = Food Standards Agency (**www.fsascience.net/2008/05/06/baby_bottle_safety**)
6. EFSA = European Food Safety Authority (**www.efsa.europa.eu/EFSA/efsa_locale-1178620753812_1178710289744.htm**)
7. The NTP = National Toxicology Program (**www.niehs.nih.gov/health/docs/bpa-factsheet.pdf**)
8. **www.medpagetoday.com/Dermatology/8927**
9. Stockholm Convention on Persistent Organic Pollutants, Stockholm, 22 May 2001, (**www.pops.int/documents/signature/signstatus.htm**)
10. See reference 46

SECTION 2: THE "BODY BURDEN" OF CHEMICALS AND THOSE MOST COMMONLY PRESENT IN THE TISSUES

Table 1 (above), only lists **some** of the **most likely**, potentially toxic, chemicals that we may be exposed to. It does not include hair dyes, Teflon coatings (perfluorinated compounds, PFCs) of cooking pans, heavy metals such a tin, lead and mercury, or any of the other thousands of other chemicals registered with the EU.

Many of these chemicals will be broken down by the liver while others will remain and accumulate in the body for many years to form the **Body Burden.**

ALTHOUGH IT IS DIFFICULT TO PROVE BEYOND DOUBT, it is reasonable to assume that, after a certain point, the Body Burden may become toxic and contribute to disease (see, Section 4, below).

- **It is also most important to understand that foetuses in the womb, babies and rapidly developing children are likely to be more sensitive to chemical contaminants than are adults.**

- For example, **thyroid hormones (eg. thyroxine)** play key roles in foetal brain development, and contaminants, such as PCBs, may decrease thyroxine levels and disrupt normal foetal brain development.

- These contaminants **can be passed on to the foetus** and baby via the mother's milk at all stages of development. They can also adversely affect the foetus **well below** levels described as "safe" in the adult woman.

Of the 12 groups of chemicals listed in Table 1 (above), it is important to know which ones accumulate in the body and therefore could potentially by themselves, or by interacting with others, over time, produce disease.

A number of **BIOMONITORING STUDIES (= tests on body tissues over several years)** have been or are being carried out to detect the presence and levels of chemical contaminants in the blood, urine, fat, breast milk and other tissues of people.

One of the largest studies is the Canadian Health Measures Survey of 5,000 volunteers using biomonitoring tests for 60 chemicals and heavy metals which is being carried out over a number of cycles beginning in 2007 and continuing into 2011 and beyond (see reference 47).

Other studies by the Centers for Disease Control (USA) Biomonitoring and Body Burden Reports are also ongoing. Report Number 3, 2005, measured 148 chemicals in the blood or urine collected from 2,400 people. It showed in the USA that levels of some harmful substances, including lead, dioxin, DDT and mercury, were declining. On the other hand, phthalate levels (from plastics) generally remained the same over several years with higher levels in women and 6-11 year old children (see reference 48).

In addition, other studies of human **Body Burdens** have identified contaminant chemicals remaining in the tissues where they can potentially cause harm. These studies include:

1. The World Wildlife Fund (WWF) – UK, National Biomonitoring Survey, 2003 (see reference 49)

2. The Environmental Working Group, Human Toxome Project, 2007 (see reference 50)

1. **The WWF Survey (UK)** analysed human blood serum from 155 volunteers, all of whom were 18yr or older, for levels of contaminant chemicals. A large range of well-known Persistent Organic Pollutants (POPs) were tested for including PCBs, pesticides and flame retardants (see Table 1). **The results showed that the people had, on average, 27 different chemicals in their blood** and that:

- PCBs were commonly present but levels were significantly lower than in previous surveys.

- DDT and HCH were the predominant pesticides present but their levels too were significantly lower than in previous surveys.

- There was widespread presence of the PBDE flame retardants.

- The source of the PCBs and pesticides was thought to be food while the flame retardants may have been from house dust.

2. In the Environmental Working Group, Human Toxome Project, 2007, up to 532 different contaminant chemicals were tested for in the blood, urine, or breast milk of 174 American people from babies in the uterus or newborn, teens, adults and seniors (over 65 yr) and:

- The chemicals detected included many of those described in Table 1 (above) such as pesticides, parabens, PAHs, bisphenol, PBDE, PCBs and dioxins, as well as many other contaminants including PFCs, lead, mercury etc. The presence of dioxins, mercury, PFCs and PCBs in the newborns is of concern.

In conclusion, we have a good indication that many groups of chemical contaminants find their way into the human body where they may remain and could potentially contribute to disease.

SECTION 3: EVIDENCE FOR A SYNERGISTIC (i.e. INTERACTIVE) EFFECT OF THESE CHEMICALS ON THE BODY

This section discusses opposing scientific views of synergism so if you just wish to know the basic conclusions go to page 128 and Section 5, below.

Studies **are extremely difficult to design** to test for the possible increase in toxicity of contaminants resulting from their interaction in the body with each other, i.e. **the Cocktail Effect.** This is because:

i. Mixtures of contaminants present in the environment vary greatly and also vary between different populations of people. For example, rural versus city dwellers or babies versus senior citizens will be exposed to differing cocktails of chemicals in their food and air (see reference 50).

ii. Any interactions between contaminants would be complex since the chemicals may have different targets in the body, may be broken down or stored differently and may activate or inhibit each other.

iii. We know from biomonitoring (see Section 2, above) that mixtures of contaminants commonly occur in people. However, most reports on the effects of mixtures of chemical come from studies on animals or from laboratory experiments. Information on humans is limited as experiments with people are strictly controlled.

iv. Finally, levels of contaminants in mixtures are often very low, making assessment of their impact even more difficult.

OPINIONS ABOUT THE COCKTAIL EFFECT USUALLY FALL INTO ONE OF TWO CONTRASTING GROUPS:

1. The official "independent Government" opinion represented by the Food Standards Agency (FSA). This agency confirms that there is evidence for exposure of people to mixtures of chemicals but concludes that **there is only limited evidence for any adverse effects of such combinations** (see references 51, 52).

2. Many other groups, that are independent of governments and supported by members, including the World Wildlife Fund (WWF)-UK (www.wwf.org.uk), the Environmental Working Group (EWG) (www.ewg.org), and the Pesticide Action Network (PAN) (www.pan-uk.org), believe that **the cocktail effect is extremely serious and urgent action is required.**

SO WHO SHOULD YOU BELIEVE?

- The Food Standards Agency (FSA) commissioned a report by the Committee on Toxicity on a "Risk Assessment of Mixtures of Pesticides and Similar Substances". This 2002 report, was extremely detailed, nearly 300 pages long, and considered all aspects of risks from chemical mixes. It reviewed previous scientific papers on the toxic effects of chemical mixtures, mainly pesticides and veterinary medicines. In most cases, **it was concluded that there was, for one reason or another, very little evidence for enhanced effects of mixtures** (see references 51, 52). This report was produced by extremely well-qualified scientists although the links that some members had with chemical/pharmaceutical companies are noted.

- The FSA's view seems to coincide with that of the American Chemistry Council (ACC) who pointed out that each day, as we breathe air or eat, our bodies absorb a mixture of low level natural and man-made chemicals (see reference 53). All life's activities are fuelled by chemical reactions and therefore it is not surprising that as the sensitivity of biomonitoring increases more and more chemicals will be detected at lower and lower concentrations. The potential for harm or toxicity will be determined very much by **the dose and exposure time** of these chemicals. Even natural chemicals can be toxic at high enough doses but most chemicals can be dealt with by the body at low doses. **The ACC therefore believes that we must not be too concerned about these low dose mixtures of chemicals.**

- However, the opposing view of the WWF, EWG and PAN, **that even at low levels, individual or cocktails of chemicals are potentially harmful**, has some significant supporting evidence. For example:

i. WWF points out that **there is very good evidence from wildlife to show just how harmful some of these contaminants, including pesticides, can be.** Even at low levels in the blood, they can accumulate in the fat tissues. For example, there are many accounts that the pesticide, DDT, resulted in the thinning of the eggshells of birds of prey (although this is disputed) and subsequent declines in populations of these birds in the UK, and that PCBs have seriously affected seal immunity (see reference 54). Both of these chemicals accumulate in humans too (see Biomonitoring in Section 2, above). Ok, this is not evidence for chemical interaction in a cocktail but illustrates that low levels of contaminants accumulate in tissues and may be harmful.

SO WHY SHOULD THERE NOT ALSO BE AN EFFCT IN HUMANS, NOT JUST FROM THESE TWO BANNED CHEMICALS, BUT FROM OTHERS ACCUMULATING SINGLY OR IN MIXTURES TOO?

ii. There are now also more recent reports, since the FSA study in 2002, supporting the idea that cocktails of chemicals can interact and have enhanced toxic effects.

● For example, it has been shown in the laboratory that **combinations of commonly used food additives are much more toxic when added to mouse nerve cells than what would be expected from the sum of the toxicity of the individual food additives.** This synergistic toxic effect represents about a 3 fold increase in toxicity than expected just from the toxicity of the individual additives added together. The combinations of additives used showing this synergistic toxic (interactive) effect were monosodium glutamate, brilliant blue and aspartame with quinoline yellow (see Chapter 5, Tables 1 and 3). The doses of additives used were about the same as would occur in the blood after a child had a snack and a drink (see reference 55).

● **Another simpler example of chemical interaction resulted from the discovery of the cancer–forming chemical, benzene, in soft drinks.** The benzene resulted from the interaction of the preservative, sodium benzoate, with vitamin C in the drinks. A FSA survey showed that about 30% of 150 soft drinks tested in the UK contained benzene and levels were sufficiently high to result in removal of 4 of these from sale (see reference 56). This example is important as it shows an interaction between a potential toxin, sodium benzoate, with a safe vitamin to produce a totally unexpected highly carcinogenic substance, benzene. What other surprises await discovery in chemical cocktails?

• **There are many other examples of the cocktail effect including studies on wildlife of mixtures of chemicals found in aquatic habitats.** Thus, exposure of salmon to mixtures of organophosphate and carbamate pesticides, which are commonly found in rivers, resulted in significantly higher levels of brain enzyme damage than would be expected just by addition of the toxicity of the two individual pesticides alone (see reference 57). The levels of pesticides used were similar to those found in the natural habitats of salmon. These results are relevant to mammals, too, as they have the same brain enzymes targeted by the pesticides above.

CONCLUSION

REDUCE YOUR BODY BURDEN OF CHEMICALS

Since evidence is now increasing indicating that:

- Low levels of contaminants can accumulate in tissues of the body and then cause toxic effects

- Contaminants can sometimes produce significantly higher levels of toxicity in combinations than that resulting from simple addition of the toxicity of the chemicals used alone. For example, if 10% of animals were killed by each chemical used by itself then when two were used in combination killing was not 20% but 50% or more i.e. a 30% Cocktail Effect

SECTION 4: POSSIBLE HARMFUL EFFECTS OF THE "BODY BURDEN" OF CHEMICALS AND THEIR LINK TO ONSET OF DISEASE

- In most Western countries, the incidences of breast, testicular and prostrate cancer, asthma, allergies, birth defects, low sperm counts, early puberty, behavioural and learning problems, cardiovascular disease, obesity and diabetes are on the increase.

- No doubt some, but not all, of these increases have resulted from improvements in diagnostic techniques and from various national campaigns to enhance screening for breast, prostrate and bowel cancers.

- Other factors, however, must be accounting for some of these increases in human disease since conditions, such as breast cancer and testicular cancer, have doubled in the UK since 1984 and 1975, respectively (see reference 58).

- In addition, over the last 20 years, the incidence of allergic disease has increased dramatically worldwide. In England alone, anaphylaxis (extremely rapid and dangerous allergic reaction to peanuts, bee stings etc) has increased by 51% from 2001 to 2005 (see reference 59).

- Since the development of any disease results from a complex interplay between genetics, age, nutrition, socioeconomic factors and exposure to environmental chemicals (see reference 60) then one or more of these factors must be having an enhanced influence on disease incidence.

- **Nobody knows the precise relative importance** of these factors in disease development but it is accepted that environmental factors play an important role in the development of some diseases. One estimate is that 5-13% of human health problems are environmentally related (see reference 60).

- There is, however, considerable disagreement as to the relative importance of the Body Burden of chemicals in disease production with many people believing that **DEFINITIVE PROOF HAS YET TO BE PROVIDED** (see, the American Chemistry Council – Section 3, above).

- However, biomonitoring has revealed the presence of a mixture of toxic chemicals in the human body some of which have been shown to have **serious** impacts on wildlife populations of birds and mammals and fish (see, section 2, above). These chemicals include the persistent organic pollutants (POPs, Table 1) which have been shown to result in reproductive disorders, malformations and immune deficiency in wildlife at levels comparable to those in humans (see reference 60).

- There is particular concern regarding the many endocrine (hormone) disrupting chemicals (detailed in Table 1) that may affect foetal development, sperm count, onset of puberty and be linked to cancers sensitive to hormones. Even the unborn baby may be exposed to these via the mother's milk. These same chemicals have been shown to cause hormone disruption in wildlife and may therefore also affect humans similarly. Hormones normally act at very low levels so that even low levels of these artificial hormone mimics in the human body may have significant effects (see reference 60).

- It is also generally recognised that persistent organic pollutants (POPs) in Table 1, disrupt brain development in human foetuses and babies. PCBs, in particular, are linked to impaired learning and may affect movement and reflexes in children (see reference 60).

- Mixtures of azo dye food colourants have also been shown to increase hyperactivity in children (see Chapter 5, Section 3), and sulphites have been included among the top 10 substances causing allergies.

- The quality of air inside houses may also be a source of health problems such as asthma, allergies, cancer in children (see reference 60) and adults. Chemicals found include PCBs, flame retardants and carcinogens, such as formaldehyde, from furnishings, paints and cleaners.

- There is evidence too that some childhood cancers are associated with exposure of the parents to pesticides and PAHs. These could be passed on to the foetus and baby via the mother's milk and induce mutations in these most susceptible and rapidly developing stages.

CONCLUSION

THERE'S NO SMOKE WITHOUT FIRE

REDUCE YOUR BODY BURDEN OF CHEMICALS

SECTION 5: AVOIDANCE AND REDUCTION OF BODY BURDEN OF CHEMICALS AND DETOX STRATEGIES

A number of basic steps can be followed to reduce your Body Burden of contaminants. The following are just **suggestions** that can be followed, a few at a time, depending on your situation, for example, if you or your children suffer from allergies and wish to reduce your chemical exposure.

TO AVOID PESTICIDES

- Buy some organic fruit and vegetables. It is **not necessary or possible to buy everything organic** and the most important fruit and vegetables to buy are listed at the end of Chapter 4. Many fruits and vegetables that are peeled before eating have the lowest pesticide levels. Always wash fruit and vegetables in running water even if "ready washed" is written on the packaging.

- Many organic items are not regularly available or are too expensive in UK supermarkets in which case concentrate on buying organic **potatoes, bread, cereals, porridge** and **dairy,** which are usually available.

- Use pesticides/fungicides/herbicides around the home only if absolutely necessary. Do not follow popular gardening articles that may tell you to spray regularly. A few blighted potatoes are better than people breathing in or coming into contact with powerful toxins.

- Trim off excess fat from meat and skin from poultry as these may contain accumulated pesticides.

TO REDUCE ADDITIVES IN FOOD AND DRINK

- The easiest way of avoiding additives is to drink water or pure fruit juices and NOT soft drinks of any sort, buy fresh fruit and vegetables grown locally and read food labels to find out what chemical additives you are eating. **Refer to "Summary and how to reduce additives in your diet" at the end of Chapter 5**.

- Unborn babies and young children with rapidly developing bodies will be **particularly vulnerable** to any harmful effects of additives.

- Trimming fat from meat and eating low fat dairy produce reduce dioxin intake.

TAKE CARE WITH PLASTICS

- Get rid of any polycarbonate baby bottles (usually marked with no.7 in triangle on bottom of bottles) as they may contain Bisphenol A (BPA).

- Never heat or microwave or wash in a dishwasher any plastic baby bottles.

- Use glass containers to heat baby food.

- Avoid canned food for babies and limit use in adults.

- Throw (recycle!) your plastic water bottles and do not reuse repeatedly.

- Do not store food for long periods in PVC wrap but use cellulose bags. Scrape off a thin layer of cheese stored in PVC before eating.

REDUCE THE CHEMICALS IN YOUR HEALTH AND BEAUTY PRODUCTS

- Sit down and read all the labels on your soaps, shampoos, toothpaste, exfoliants, body, hand and face creams, sunscreens, hair sprays and dyes, deodorants, shaving cream, lipstick, nail polish, perfumes etc. The list reads **like a chemical warfare mix** and not something that you expose your body to every day! See Table 1 of this Chapter for possible effects of these chemicals on your body.

- Maybe you suffer from allergies and maybe the chemicals in these products are making you worse?

- Ok, so you think that you cannot possibly go without any of these. However, what you can do is to note the main toxins present and try and buy products free of these (see references 61 and 62 for suppliers, and 63 for a safety review of cosmetics).

- From Table 1 you will see that there are **5 chemicals** in these products that are particularly important to try and eliminate:

    1. Sodium lauryl sulphate (SLS or SDS) found in many liquid soaps (washing up liquids are particularly bad due to frequency of use) and shampoos, and causing dermatitis or allergic rhinitis (runny nose and sneezing).

    2/3. The **phalates, such as DBP and DEHP,** and **parabens** (methyl- ,ethyl-, propyl- and butyl- parabens), which are hormone disruptors. In the USA, the blood and urine of 20 teenage girls tested were found to contain parabens, as well as phalates in some (see reference 64).

    4/5. The **polyethylene glycols (PEGs)** and **propylene glycol** that are irritants or contain carcinogens.

- As an example, you can buy "Simple Soap" without any of these 5 chemicals and also without fragrances which can also be a problem.

REDUCE CHEMICALS/IRRITANTS IN THE HOUSE

- It is very difficult to do this as the average house has many sources of contaminant chemicals in everyday products.

- Have fun with the children and check out the toxic chemicals in a typical house (see reference 65).

- Buy more natural or environmentally safe cleaning agents (see reference 66) which are available for the toilet, washing up and for cleaning surfaces. Avoid "antibacterial" products (creating superbugs?) and always wear gloves when cleaning or washing up.

- Do not use insect sprays indoors.

- Use natural air fresheners like bunches of lavender in draws and cupboards.

- Avoid scented detergents/conditioners in the laundry.

- Use shoe cleaners outside with gloves on.

- Furnishings, carpets and mattresses will be treated with chemicals so try and find out what these are and decide if you want these in your home. Keep the rooms well aerated if possible and leave plastic covers in place for a while if possible. In particular, avoid flame retardants (PBDE) which are now banned in the EU.

- Store paints and cleaners well away from main living areas.

- If you are highly allergic, use house dust mite proof covers on bed linen.

- Vacuum clean regularly to reduce dust laden with household chemicals. Do not forget to vacuum the curtains.

- Use glass, stainless steel or cast iron cooking vessels rather than non-stick and Teflon-coated.

- Avoid dry cleaning clothes due to toxic solvents used.

DETOX, ESPECIALLY IF YOU ARE TRYING FOR A BABY

- The Body Burden of chemicals will continue to accumulate unless at least some of the above steps are followed to reduce the so-called **"Toxic Load"**. It makes sense to prevent further build up of contaminants which will subsequently be released into the body over many years.

- Normally, the body is extremely efficient at removing most toxins taken in but some, such as the dioxins and PCBs, accumulate in the fatty tissues. It has been estimated that some dioxins and PCBs can remain stored in the fat for 7-11 years or more (see reference 67).

- There is also a belief that the body can only accumulate a certain amount of contaminants and **above this maximal capacity** damage occurs resulting in allergies and ill health (see reference 68).

- The potential importance of reducing the Body Burden, especially for women planning a pregnancy, is illustrated by work showing **the transference of up to 69% of dioxins, as well as PCBs and other chemicals, from a mother's body into the fat of her milk during nursing of her baby** over a two year period (see reference 69).

- The Schecter study, however, is not scientifically significant as it only looked at one nursing mother and urgently needs repeating (see reference 69). There is also much debate as to whether these contaminants might cause harm to the baby.

- Finally, there are those who advocate active detox programmes to reduce the Body Burden as these have been shown to be successful. For example, following the collapse of the World Trade Centre, police, firemen, paramedics and labourers were exposed to high levels of PCBs and dioxins which accumulated at elevated levels in their bodies. A detoxification programme was undertaken and some significant reductions of pollutants were recorded which resulted in adverse health symptoms returning to normal (see reference 70).

- The value and safety, however, of such detox programmes are the subject of much debate. Some organisations are offering detox treatments which are not necessarily based upon sound and proven scientific and medical proof.

- The best approach is to reduce your Body Burden, as outlined above, making sure that you adopt a balanced diet (see Chapter 1) to control your weight, and participate in a regular exercise programme (see Chapters 9-11).

- Some additional references to detox methods, food and cosmetic additives as well as toxins in the environment are provided for those particularly concerned (see references 71-75).

CHAPTER 7

VITAMINS AND SUPPLEMENTS - 1

THE "TAKE OR NOT TAKE" DILEMMA

i. What evidence indicates the need for vitamins and supplements?

ii. What "goodness" is left in our food after processing?

iii. Tables of vitamins and supplements including functions and doses.

"To Take Or Not To Take That Is The Question?"

ARE YOU CONFUSED as to whether or not to take supplements? No wonder, just look at some of the news headlines that have appeared and have done much to add to our confusion:

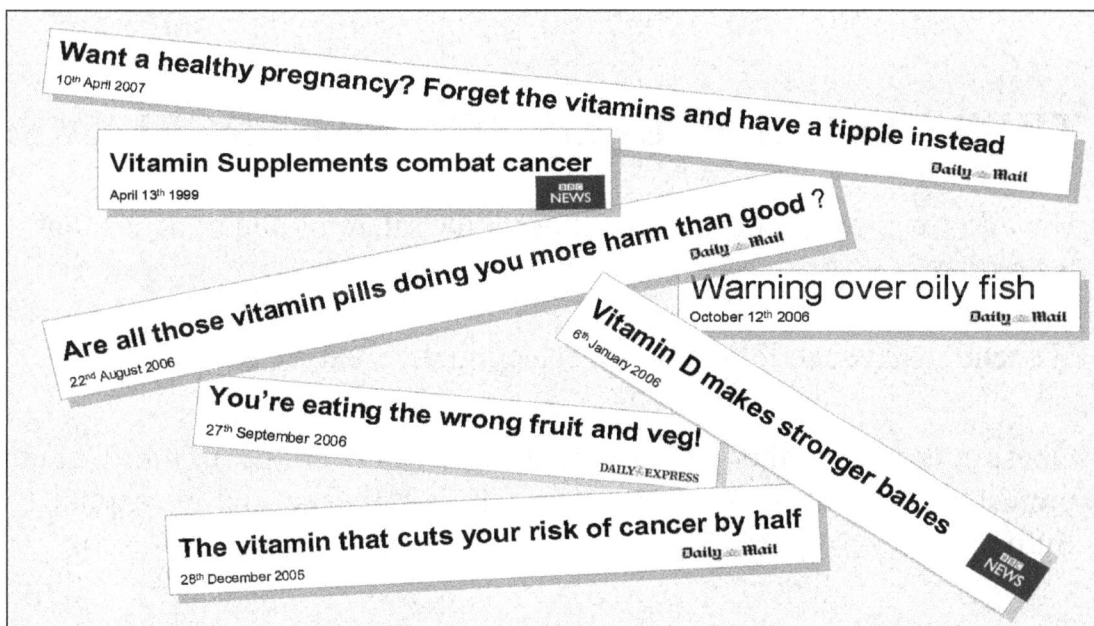

Want a healthy pregnancy? Forget the vitamins and have a tipple instead
10th April 2007
Daily Mail

Vitamin Supplements combat cancer
April 13th 1999
BBC NEWS

Are all those vitamin pills doing you more harm than good?
Daily Mail
22nd August 2006

Warning over oily fish
October 12th 2006
Daily Mail

You're eating the wrong fruit and veg!
27th September 2006
DAILY EXPRESS

Vitamin D makes stronger babies
6th January 2006
BBC NEWS

The vitamin that cuts your risk of cancer by half
Daily Mail
28th December 2005

Many such articles appear almost daily in newspapers, magazines and books **advocating the use of dietary supplements** while doctors and many nutritionists recommend obtaining all necessary vitamins and minerals from a **"healthy balanced diet"**.

What exactly is a "healthy balanced diet"?

As described in Chapter 1 (pages 26-28), a balanced diet would include a combination of foods from all the main food groups (below) at each meal. Thus, in theory, the balanced diet should provide all our daily requirements of vitamins and minerals.

1. **Bread, cereals, pasta, rice or potatoes** i.e., high in carbohydrate or "starchy" foods.

2. **Fruit and vegetables** (at least 5 per portions per day – see Chapter 1) for healthy carbohydrate, protein (pulses), fibre and vitamins.

3. **Meat as a source of protein** to include red meat, poultry, fish, eggs, or meat substitutes such as nuts and pulses (peas, beans and lentils). Avoid too much red meat (beef, pork, ham, lamb) i.e. not every day.

4. **Milk and dairy products** to include milk, cheese and yoghurt (all low-fat or skimmed) to provide some protein but also calcium and B vitamins.

THERE ARE, HOWEVER, SEVERAL PROBLEMS:

- How do we know if our food contains all the vitamins and minerals that we require?

- We tend to have too little time for selecting the food we eat.

- Obesity levels in the UK are soaring with over 12 million adults projected to be obese by 2010. The UK is now the obesity capital of Europe.

- There are about 3 million people in the UK suffering from malnutrition.

CONCLUSIONS

1. Obviously, a huge number of people in the UK do not have a balanced diet. It is therefore unhelpful for the medical experts to repeatedly advise that "vitamin and mineral supplements are not required if you have a balanced diet".

2. Processed or convenience foods are the main culprits responsible for producing obesity and poorly balanced diets. There is also concern over the poor diet of 15-21 year olds, many of whom are also at risk of malnutrition (see reference 76). In addition, of the estimated 3 million malnourished people in the UK, a large number are **elderly and are at particular risk in care homes and hospitals** (see reference 77).

There is also concern about:

THE NUTRITIONAL VALUE OF OUR FOOD

- Even if we adopt an apparently balanced diet what guarantee do we have that our food is providing all the essential vitamins and minerals required?

- Problems with the nutritional content of our food have been highlighted for some years but mainly ignored. Joanne Blythman has researched this topic extensively in her books entitled "The Food We Eat" (1996) and "Bad Food Britain" (2006) (references 78, 79).

- Basically, as a Nation, we shop for food in supermarkets due to time constraints and the convenience of finding everything we need in one location. The problem is that as a result we are hooked on convenience foods that are often **highly processed with their nutritional value degraded**.

- It is true that the supermarkets stock "fresh" fruit and vegetables but many of these are foreign in origin and harvested days or weeks previously with the loss of vital vitamins and minerals. Apparently, **our food may now be "nutritionally impoverished"** (Blythman, 2006, reference 79).

WHAT IS FOOD PROCESSING?

This includes all the stages the food goes through before it is eaten. Processing thus involves the treatment during growing such as spraying with pesticides, as well as special techniques that the food subsequently goes through before eating including milling, preservation, storage, transportation and cooking, all of which will partially degrade the vitamin and mineral content of the food.

a. Growing - Conventional Farming Versus Organic Farming

- Most of our food crops are grown by intensive farming with the aid of synthetic fertilizers. According to the **Food Standards Agency (FSA)**, the **nutritional content of these foods is no less** than crops grown organically (see reference 80). The FSA was set up by the Government to protect public health in relation to food.

- **The FSA's conclusion contrasts the view of the Soil Association (SA)**, a charitable organization independent of Government and concerned with promoting organic food and farming, which concluded (see reference 81) that organic food had higher levels of vitamin C, as well as of other antioxidants and essential minerals.

- The SA's conclusion was based on a review of 41 studies from around the World and included evidence that between the years of 1941 and 1991, trace elements (=dietary components, such as copper, iron, selenium, and zinc, present only in minute quantities in our food but essential for maintaining health, see Table 2, below) **in conventionally grown fruit and vegetables had fallen by 76%.**

- Clearly, the debate concerning the nutritional values of conventional versus organically grown foods has some way to run and requires more scientific examination. Unfortunately, the FSA's view may be questioned as it is a Government related agency (remember BSE and the "healthy hamburger") while the SA, it could also be argued, is also biased in favour of organic food.

- **Recently, however, a 18 million euros, EU-funded project, showed that organic vegetables (including potatoes, carrots, cabbage and lettuce) and fruit contain up to 40 percent more antioxidants (such as vitamin C) than conventionally-farmed produce. Organic milk was also found to contain 60 percent more antioxidants (such as vitamin E) and beneficial fatty acids, including omega 3. In addition, organic food was shown to contain lower levels of pesticides and heavy metals. The research was included in the EU "Quality Low Imput Food (QLIF)" project and lead by Professor Carlo Leifert. The research involved over 31 institutes, companies and universities and took place over 5 years from March 2004 to April 2009. Most important too was the fact that to achieve these results good agricultural practices were required and details of these were included in the reports (See, www.qlif.org for leaflets and links).**

- Controversially, the FSA commissioned a report on organic versus conventionally produced food, published in 2009, which concluded that although differences exist between these foods, they were "not large enough to be of any public health significance" (see references 82, 83). The FSA study seems to have ignored the Leifert reports (www.qlif.org) although details were being released of these in 2007.

WHO SHOULD THE POOR CONFUSED PUBLIC BELIEVE?

- The FSA report was not an original experimental study but a review of previously published work. The analyses included the results from studies published several decades ago probably before the best agricultural practices had been developed for organic food. The importance of such best practice was emphasized by Leifert and colleagues (see, www.qlif.org).

- In contrast to the FSA review, the Leifert QLIF reports were based on large scale, original experimental studies actually growing crops and rearing animals under optimised conventional and organic conditions.

- There has been widespread criticism of the FSA report for ignoring the QLIF reports.

- Until the FSA considers the QLIF reports objectively and gives reasons for rejecting such important research, then it is logical to accept the findings of the extremely comprehensive QLIF study.

- In addition, most importantly, **many people buy organic food not because of nutritional advantages, but because of the lower levels of pesticide residues in organic food**. The FSA even supports this point of view.

Many people already believe that organic food:

Tastes better

Has increased nutrient content

Undoubtedly has reduced contamination with pesticides

Has environmental benefits that preserve and encourage wildlife as a result of the use of fewer chemicals and intercropping

Other people point out that with organic food:

Carbon emissions may be much higher as so much is imported

Since yields are lower, more land is required for growing crops

There are reports, for example in chickens, that organic food has higher contamination rates with harmful microorganisms

If you decide to opt for organic food then do this very selectively (see Chapter 4 for details of which organic foods to choose) to avoid wasting money.

b. Growing - Use of Pesticides

This is, of course, part of the growing process but deserves some separate consideration due to the possible involvement of pesticide residues in the development of human disease. There is now evidence to show that about 30% of our basic conventionally grown foods contain pesticide residues (see Tables 1 to 3 in Chapter 4) but the effect of these residues on our health is debatable (discussed in detail in Chapter 6). Two things, however, are clear:

i. Our bodies contain cocktails of chemical pollutants derived from pesticides in our food, from worming agents in our livestock, from chemicals contaminating the air we breathe and from products we use on our bodies or in our homes (see details in Chapter 6 "The Cocktail Effect"). These chemicals may interact in the body to compromise our health.

ii. We must not, due to our fear of chemical contamination, **completely stop eating** vegetables and fruit grown conventionally. The benefits of the "five a day" policy must far outweigh the harm resulting from a diet free of vegetables and fruit. Again, refer to Chapter 4 "Is Our Food Safe?" for selecting foods with the lowest pesticide contamination levels.

c. Milling – OUR OBSESSION WITH WHITE BREAD AND RICE

- White flour and white rice are made by **removing the outer layers of the wheat or rice seeds** using special milling machines. This produces the white flour for making white bread and pasta, as well as the polished white rice that most people buy.

- We have been brainwashed into thinking that anything white is superior and healthy but this is simply not true. **The outer layers of the wheat and rice seeds contain over 90% of the bran and most of the vitamins and minerals.**

Figure 1. Showing wholemeal and white loaves and the possible advantages and disadvantages of eating each type of bread

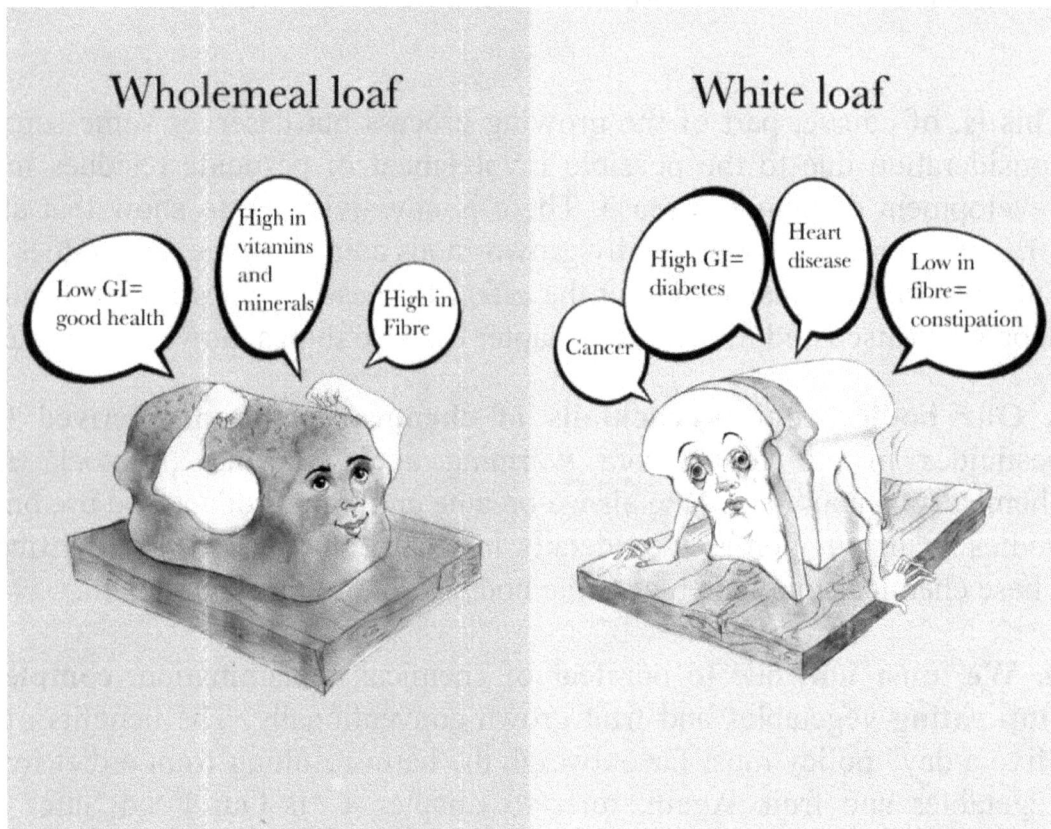

- Generally speaking, white flour is worse for us than white rice simply because white flour is also subjected to **bleaching with toxic chemicals**.

- **Thus, white flour is devoid of essential nutrients and is usually eaten by people who subsequently suffer with higher rates of heart disease, some cancers and type II diabetes (i.e. not dependent on insulin injections but treated by diet and exercise, see reference 84, for example).**

- Just think of the number of biscuits and cakes on the supermarket shelves that have been made with white flour. Even white bread "fortified" with added synthetic vitamins and nutrients is not nearly as good as bread (organic) made from wholemeal or whole grains. White rice, however, does still contain some protein, vitamins and minerals.

Figure 2. Wholemeal and whole grain loaves

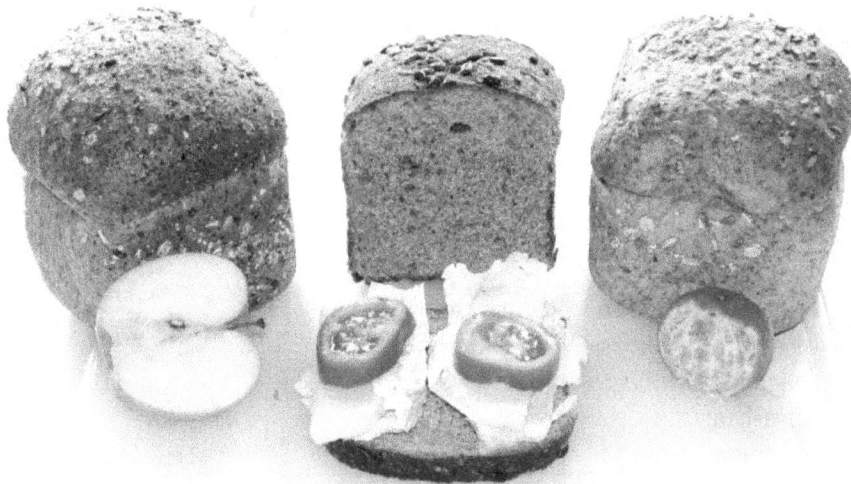

d. Preservation and Storage

These are necessary in order to prevent breakdown of the food by microbes and enzymes so it can be stored and transported before use. There are many preservation techniques and the main advantages and disadvantages of the various methods are shown below in Table 1.

Table 1.   ADVANTAGES AND DISADVANTAGES OF MAIN METHODS USED TO PRESERVE FOOD

Preservation method	Advantages	Disadvantages
Refrigeration and freezing	Good for nutrient preservation	Slow loss of nutrients, blanching reduces levels of some vitamins
Canning (tinned food)	Food can be stored at room temperature for long periods	Loss of water-soluble nutrients eg. vitamin C, riboflavin, thiamine into canning fluid
Smoking and curing mainly of meat and fish	Dries, flavours and preserves food	Smoked food may be linked to stomach and other cancers
Drying mainly of fruits, meats, fish, cereals, soup, coffee	Removes water prevents microbial growth and stops enzymes that breakdown food	Sulphites sometimes added to dried fruit may cause allergies. Limited loss of vitamin B and C
Chemical additives includes nitrites, nitrates, sulphur dioxide, benzoates etc.	Improves shelf life, appearance and taste of food and inhibits microbial growth and poisoning	Linked to cancer formation, allergies, fertility problems, and adverse children's behavior – see Chapters 5 and 6
Heat sterilisation of milk and juices (pasteurization and ultra-heat treatment, UHT)	Long shelf life at room temperature	Loss of some nutrients but less than in in canning
Added salt or sugar eg. meats and jams	Good for nutrient preservation	High salt content associated with high blood pressure
Irradiation of limited use and mainly for spices and condiments in UK	Prolongs shelf life, killing insects and bacteria, delays fruit ripening and sprouting in vegetables	Some safety concerns and loss of nutrients including antioxidants*

* See details in reference 85

THE CONCLUSION from Table 1, above, is that all preservation methods either result in the loss of vitamins or minerals or else may result in concerns about health safety. Obviously, for maximizing our intake of vitamins and minerals, we should all be eating recently harvested/killed foodstuffs. In our modern, fast-paced, society this is clearly impossible all the time. The secret is to compromise and be aware of the shortcomings of the modern diet and whenever possible to introduce locally grown, fresh food. Failing this, then frozen foods are acceptable with limited nutrient loss and few if any chemical additives.

e. Food Transportation

- Transportation of food leads to a **significant loss of vital nutrients**, the extent of which will depend upon the time and distance travelled. In the USA, it has been estimated that the components of a basic meal have travelled 1500 miles to arrive at the dinner plate.

- Many of the numerous fruits and vegetables on display in supermarkets throughout the year in the UK have also travelled thousands of miles to arrive on the shelves.

- In addition, with green vegetables, the entire marketing route from harvesting, blanching, freezing, transportation, storage, distribution, purchase and consumption has been estimated to take about 60 days (see reference 86). During this time, spinach, beans and peas all lose significant amounts of vitamin C, which reaches more than a 50 percent loss with spinach.

- Remember much organic produce is also imported and has thus undergone significant nutrient loss thus cancelling out one important benefit, i.e. higher vitamin content, of buying organic food.

- Locally purchased, non-organic, fruit and vegetables will probably match organic produce for nutrient content although the other benefits of organic, such as reduced pesticide contamination, will still apply. The optimum is to buy locally grown organic food, not only for the nutritional advantages, but also to reduce the carbon emissions from transportation which results in global warming.

f. Cooking

Inevitably, cooking food leads to a further loss of nutrients but this will depend upon:

- **The method of cooking** with boiling in excess hot water leading to the loss of many water-soluble vitamins such as vitamins B and C and minerals including calcium. A study on the effect of different cooking methods on the antioxidant content of freshly picked broccoli showed that microwaving, boiling and pressure cooking resulted in 47 to 97 percent loss of antioxidants while **steamed broccoli was similar to the raw vegetable in antioxidant content** (see reference 87). Microwaving, however, was shown by the same authors to be far less damaging to the nutrient content of vegetables if the amount of water used for cooking was kept to a minimum.

- **The temperature and the length of the cooking time** which if too high/long will result in further nutrient loss. This is particularly a problem in cafeterias where food is often kept hot for too long under bright lights.

- **The type of food cooked** with, for example, rice rapidly losing vitamins and minerals unless washed and cooked in minimal volumes of water. In contrast, eggs lose few nutrients during cooking.

- **The nutrient involved** with water-soluble vitamins B and C rapidly lost by boiling while fat-soluble vitamins such as vitamin A are more resistant to leaching into the cooking water.

THE BASIC RULES FOR RETAINING THE MAXIMAL NUTRIENT CONTENT OF FOOD DURING COOKING ARE:

1. Steam food for the minimal time

2. If you boil or microwave then cover the food to retain the steam and speed up the cooking process

3. Use the minimal water for cooking, especially for rice

4. Use the cooking or steaming water as a stock for sauces and stews

5. Do not soak food before cooking i.e. do not prepare the vegetables the previous day and store in water

6. Do not keep the cooked food hot for long but eat as soon as possible

7. Eat some freshly prepared uncooked fruit/vegetables every day

COOKING – IT'S NOT ALL BAD NEWS

Cooking not only makes food more palatable but also kills off harmful microbes. In addition, it releases from the cells of fruit and vegetables higher concentrations of antioxidants such as lycopene for absorption in the gut. Lycopene has multiple benefits in preventing prostate cancer and cardiovascular disease (see Chapter 1).

WHAT IS THE EVIDENCE THAT WE NEED TO TAKE VITAMINS AND OTHER SUPPLEMENTS?

1. From the section above on food processing, it is obvious that in many cases there may be serious depletion of essential nutrients, such as vitamins and minerals in food.

2. Recent studies do indicate that certain key nutrients are at too low levels in our diet.

3. We also know that there are about 3 million people, many of whom are elderly, suffering malnutrition in the UK. Most of these would probably benefit from supplements.

4. Research has also shown that many people have levels of vitamins in their bodies below recommended daily allowances. This topic will be discussed in Chapter 8 in detail after we have briefly listed, below (Tables 2 and 3), the main vitamins and minerals required in our diet.

Don't just plough through these Tables as they are for your reference after you have decided which supplements you need to take (see Chapter 8 "The Bottom Line")

Table 2.   FUNCTIONS AND SOURCES OF VITAMINS THAT ARE COMMONLY TAKEN AS DIETARY SUPPLEMENTS

Name ↓	RDA[1] + Deficiency Symptoms	Safe Upper Limit[2] Per day	In Which Foods	Functions To Maintain
Vitamin A (retinol, beta carotene)	0.6-0.7mg[3] Night blindness; other problems in developing countries	General use as supplement not advised, especially by smokers	Liver and fish oils, yellow/orange fruit and vegetables, leafy greens	Healthy bones, teeth, hair, eyesight, and lining of mouth, nose, lungs and reproductive system
Vitamin B1 (thiamine)	1.1-1.5 mg[3] Muscular weakness, tiredness, poor memory; alcoholics often affected	Unknown, 40 mg+?	Offal, lean meat, fish, eggs, milk, whole grain bread, cereals and pasta, brown rice	Energy release from food; brain, nerve and heart functions; prevents brain damage in alcoholics
Vitamin B2 (riboflavin)	1.1-1.3 mg[3] Sores around nose and lips; itching, sore throat; sensitivity to light	Unknown, but no more 40 mg advised	Liver, cheese, eggs, milk, green vegetables like broccoli, whole grain bread, cereals and pasta	Energy release from food; healthy skin, hair, nails, eyesight; assists adrenalin production and iron absorption

Vitamin B3 (niacin which occurs as nicotinamide and nicotinic acid)	13-17 mg[3] Eruptions on skin in sunlight; swollen tongue; insomnia and diarrhoea	Unknown but no more 35-50 mg advised	Liver, red meat, poultry and fish, whole grain bread, cereals, nuts and beans	Energy release from food; healthy skin; promotes nervous system and gut functions and sex hormone production
Vitamin B5 (pantothenic acid)	6 mg Deficiency rare and only seen with severe starvation; burning feet and restlessness	Unknown but no more 500 mg advised	Liver, kidney, chicken, beef, eggs, broccoli, whole grain bread and cereals, nuts and beans	Energy release from food; essential for growth and healthy nervous system; synthesis of hormones, red blood cells and antibodies
Vitamin B6 (pyridoxine)	No RDA but 1.2-1.6 mg[3] advised Deficiency unusual; signs are dermatitis, sore tongue, anaemia, confusion, irritability, impaired immunity	10 mg	Liver, chicken, red meat, whole grain bread and cereals, avocadoes, bananas, tuna, salmon, sunflower seeds, peanut butter	Red blood cells and haemoglobin synthesis, immune and nervous system functions, normal levels of blood sugar, absorption of vitamin B 12, production of some hormones
Vitamin B7 (biotin or vitamin H)	RDA (USA) 0.3 mg (300 µg) Deficiency rare; dermatitis, rash around eyes, exhaustion, loss of appetite, muscle pain	Unknown but no more than 0.9 mg (900 µg) advised	Liver, kidney, milk, cheese, egg yolk, nuts, bananas, broccoli, soya, whole grain bread and cereals	Hair, nails and skin? Also for energy production
Vitamin B9 (folic acid)	0.2-0.4 mg[4] (=200-400 µg) Anaemia; spina bifida in newborn babies	Unknown but no more 1 mg advised	Liver, whole grain bread and cereals, broccoli, spinach, nuts, oranges	Formation of blood cells; healthy nervous system in unborn babies
Vitamin B12 (cobalamin)	1.5 µg Pernicious anaemia, brain, nerve and heart damage	Unknown but no more 2 mg (2000 µg) advised	Animal produce-liver, meat, fish, eggs, milk, but also in soya milk and added to cereals	Formation of red blood cells; healthy nervous system
Vitamin C (ascorbic acid)	40-60 mg[3] Scurvy with bleeding gums, weakness, painful joints, anaemia, and bruising	Unknown, more than 1gram may give gut problems	Citrus fruits i.e. oranges; other fruits such as berries, kiwis; also in green leafy vegetables including spinach and broccoli	Healthy bones, teeth and gums; iron absorption and wound healing; resistance to infection due to antioxidant function

Vitamin D (calciferol)	No RDA but 10-15 μg[3] advised Failure of bone growth, and rickets in children	Unknown, but no more than 25 μg advised	Liver, dairy produce, oily fish but main source is sunlight on skin	Healthy teeth, bones, nerves, muscles and blood clotting; may reduce cancer
Vitamin E (tocopherol)	No RDA but 3-15 mg (4.5-22.5 IU) advised. Deficiency rare but may result from harmful action of oxygen radicals from cell processes or pollution such as cigarette smoke	Unknown but no more than 540 mg (800 IU) advised	Highest in vegetable oils (olive, sunflower, corn, soya); also in whole grain bread and cereals, meat, leafy greens-spinach and kale	Antioxidant activity, protecting cell membranes from oxygen radicals arising from cell processes and environmental pollution such as cigarette smoke. Prevents anaemia and, although proof incomplete, may slow aging and reduce heart attacks?
Vitamin K (phylloquinone)	No RDA but 120 μg per day sufficient. Deficiency unusual but may result from gut problems resulting in poor absorption	Unknown but no more than 1 mg advised	Liver, milk and eggs, fatty fish and fish oils, plant oils like soya and rape seed, dark leafy vegetables – spinach and broccoli	Coagulation of blood and healthy bones

1. RDA (Recommended Daily Allowances) **from all sources,** including food, drink and supplements, given for adults 18 yr + only. Children less than 18 yr require significantly lower doses (see references 88, 89).

2. Safe Upper Limit per day (SUL) (see reference 90).

3. The lower RDA is for women and the upper RDA for men.

4. 0.4mg folic acid is recommended as a supplement for pregnant women up to week 12 of pregnancy.

Table 3. FUNCTIONS AND SOURCES OF MINERALS, TRACE METALS AND SOME MISCELLANEOUS FACTORS THAT ARE COMMONLY TAKEN AS DIETARY SUPPLEMENTS

Name ↓	RDA[1] + Deficiency Symptoms	Safe Upper Limit [2] Per day	In Which Foods	Functions To Maintain
Boron	No RDA but 1.5-2 mg advised Osteoporosis in elderly?	6 mg	Nuts, fresh fruit, peas, beans and green vegetables	Healthy bones by preventing osteoporosis and arthritis by influencing calcium and magnesium balance?
Calcium	800 mg[3] Weak bones and teeth, osteoporosis, stunted growth	1,500 mg	Dairy products, nuts, salmon, sardines, green leafy vegetables like broccoli and cabbage, tofu	Healthy bones and teeth, muscle and heart functions, blood clotting, mental health (?) and may protect against breast, prostate and colon cancers?
Chromium	No RDA but at least 0.025 mg required Deficiency rare outside hospital	Unknown but no more than 10 mg advised. General use not advised	Meat, whole grain bread and cereals, pulses and spices	Insulin levels and thus influences energy obtained from food
Copper	No RDA Anaemia and bone malformation	No more than 10 mg advised	Liver, shellfish, whole grain bread, cereals, nuts	Functions of many enzymes, energy production, growth, immunity, blood cell formation, heart and brain functions
Iodine	150 µg [4] Goiter, lethargy, weakness, weight gain, lower IQ, miscarriage, stillbirth, and birth defects	No more than 500 µg Advised	Milk, cheese, turkey, marine fish, shellfish, sea salt and seaweed (kelp)	Production of thyroid hormones that regulate energy production; also required for development of brain in foetus and children

Iron	8-18 mg [5] Anaemia with associated fatigue and palpitations	Unknown but adverse effects above 50 mg	Liver, red meat, whole grain bread and cereals, oysters, pulses, dark green leafy vegetables, apricots, molasses and tofu	Oxygen transport around body, immune functions and energy production
Magnesium	300-400 mg[5] Deficiency rare but results in fatigue, as well as heart, gut, nervous and skeletal disorders	Unknown but no more than 400 mg Advised	In many foods including high levels in whole grain bread and cereals, green leafy vegetables, nuts, brown rice	Energy production, cell multiplication and cell interactions, vitamin D and hormone activities
Manganese	No RDA but Adequate Dietary Intake set at 2-5 mg for adults. Deficiency rare	Unknown but no more than 0.5 mg as a supplement?	Tea (particularly green), whole grain bread and cereals, spinach, pineapple, nuts, brown rice	Enzyme functions involved in many processes such as antioxidant activity, bone and cartilage formation, wound healing, control of blood sugar and cholesterol levels
Phosphorus	700 mg Deficiency rare and at starvation in anorexics and alcoholics	Unknown but no more than 250 mg as a supplement	Meat, poultry, fish, dairy, whole grain bread and cereals, nuts, beans, peas	Energy production, bone and tissue structure, hormone and enzyme activities
Potassium	No RDA, 3,500 mg recommended Deficiency from vomiting, diarrhoea, alcoholism, sweating, dieting, heart failure resulting in muscle weakness, fatigue, abnormal heart beat	Unknown but no more than 4900 mg	Liver, meat, fish, milk, fruit (bananas, citrus, raisins), vegetables (potatoes, spinach)	Correct internal water balance of cells and tissues that is essential for all life processes
Selenium	55 µg Deficiency in long-term hospitalized patients on artificial diets also in Crohn's disease, causes heart and joint damage	450 µg	Offal, pork, fish, whole grain bread Brazil nuts (very high levels), seeds	Antioxidant activity against harmful free radicals produced by body and may help protect against some cancers?
Sodium (chloride)	No RDA but 3-4 g recommended in adults. Deficiency rare except with excess sweating	Unknown but no more than 6 g in diet advised. Not used as supplement	Main source is from processed food and salt added at mealtimes	With potassium, determines correct internal water balance of cells and tissues as well as blood volume and pressure; also component of body secretions

Zinc	15 mg Poor growth and development, reduced immunity and wound healing, mental retardation, nerve damage, night blindness	42 mg	Oysters (very high levels), all meats, milk and cheese, cereals and bread	Immune functioning, growth and development, reproduction, many enzyme functions throughout body

SOME ADDITIONAL MISCELLANEOUS SUPPLEMENTS[6]

Aspirin	75mg (coated)	Long term use not advised unless under medical supervision	Pills	Prevention of colon and prostate cancer, heart attacks, strokes and Alzheimer's?
Co-enzyme Q10 (ubiquinone)	No RDA but 50-200 mg advised as supplement depending on disease	Unknown, no toxicity reported	Offal, oily fish, whole grain bread and cereals, peanuts and vegetable oils	Energy production, antioxidant activity, periodontal health
Fish Oils[7] (Omega-3 Fatty Acids)	No RDA but 500-1000 mg capsules usually taken containing 450 mg fatty acids. Capsules vary in content of fatty acids	Unknown, but beware cod liver oil capsules which contain high levels of vitamin A	Omega-3 fatty acids present naturally in fish, also in tofu, and soybeans, walnuts flaxseed and oils made from these but plant sources are of limited use.[7]	Healthy heart, brain development in foetus, and joint motility to reduce symptoms of arthritis. Capsules of fish oil also contain vitamin D (see benefits in Table 2, above)
Garlic	No RDA but 600-900 mg by mouth recommended	Unknown	In raw cloves, pills, powder, oil, juice syrup or tincture	Reduction of cholesterol levels. Prevention of cancer and infections? Thinning of blood and reduction of blood pressure?
Glucosamine sulphate or hydrochloride	No RDA but 1500 mg by mouth recommended	Unknown but beware of sulphate if blood pressure high	Pills/capsules	Treatment for pain and immobility of osteoarthritis

1. RDA (Recommended Daily Allowances **from all sources including food, drink and supplements**) given mainly for adults 18 yr + only. Children less than 18 yr require significantly lower doses while elderly people and pregnant women may need higher levels (see references 88, 89).

2.	Safe Upper Limit per day (SUL) (see reference 90).

3.	Higher levels of calcium (another 500 mg) may be required in breast-feeding women and additional calcium may be needed by elderly people (see Chapter 8 for details).

4.	Pregnant and breast feeding women may require iodine supplements to raise intake levels but consult your doctor. Multivitamins contain iodine.

5.	The lower iron RDA is for men and the higher RDA is for women.

6.	These supplements are included just as examples of the many other substances taken daily by people. Only garlic and coenzyme Q10 are diet related.

7.	It is better to use fish oil rather than cod liver oil supplements since the latter also have high concentrations of vitamin A which could be toxic to pregnant and elderly people. Pregnant women should also use pure sources of omega-3 such as krill as fish oils may be contaminated with heavy metals and pesticides. Plant sources of omega-3 fatty acids, such as flaxseeds, walnuts and Soya, may not be utilized as efficiently by the body as fish oils but opinions differ (see reference 91).

CHAPTER 8

VITAMINS AND SUPPLEMENTS – 2

"THE BOTTOM LINE"

In the UK population of 61.4 million, 45 million people belong to groups likely to benefit from taking vitamin/mineral supplements

What to take is explained

In a hurry? Just identify below which particular group of people you belong to and read your recommended daily vitamin and mineral supplements

Tables 2 and 3 in Chapter 7 give sources of these vitamins/ minerals in different foods and the total recommended daily allowances (RDA) of those required from food, drink and supplements

WARNING: Vitamin, mineral and herb supplements may interact with medicines (see page 186, below)

REMEMBER, whenever possible, it is better to modify your diet to obtain your vitamins *naturally*, however, many people are probably more likely to take a vitamin pill than change their diet.

SOME BASIC FACTS ABOUT THE UK POPULATION

The UK population was 61.4 million in 2008 which included 39 million 16-64 year olds of which nearly 50% were overweight (27%) or obese (23%).

The 61.4 million people can approximately be broken down into:

1. 19.6 million 16-64 yr olds of normal weight.*

2. 19.6 million 16-64 yr olds overweight or obese.

3. 9.9 million over 65 yr old.

4. 12.3 million children less than 16 yr old.

5. 3.9 million 16-64 yr olds (included in groups 1 and 2, above) who smoke and/or drink excessively (a very reserved estimate).

6. About 2 million pregnant or breast feeding women (included in groups 1, 2 and 5 (above).

*Some of these "normal" people will include, vegetarians, dieters, diabetics, anaemia sufferers, and Islamic women, all of whom will require supplements.

From the above, an estimate of the number of UK people likely to benefit from taking vitamin and mineral supplements is approximately 45 million. Only about 16 million adults have a normal weight and, hopefully, a balanced diet.

SUPPLEMENT REQUIREMENTS OF DIFFERENT GROUPS OF PEOPLE

i. "NORMAL" HEALTHY PEOPLE 19-59 YEARS OLD. The vitamin and mineral supplement market in the UK is worth about £300 million per year. Over 40% of adults take supplements with the 50-65 year olds the highest users (see reference 92). The most commonly taken supplements are cod liver oil and multivitamins. Only 2% of supplement consumers take high dose vitamin/minerals, with vitamin C as the most popular for use. Most experts agree that vitamins in supplements do not have the same effect on the body as vitamins eaten in foods. An apple, for example, not only contains vitamin C but also a complex mixture of other vitamins, antioxidants and phytochemicals which interact in the body. The action of a single supplement on the body taken as a pill in isolation will thus be very different to the mixture of vitamins/minerals in fruits or vegetables. Hence the advice from many dieticians and doctors that "**It is unnecessary for normal healthy people to take supplements as we can obtain all our vitamins/minerals from 'a balanced diet' containing at least 5 portions of fruit and vegetables per day**".

UNFORTUNATELY, according to the Foods Standards Agency National Diet & Nutrition Survey in 2004 (see reference 93), of adults aged 19 to 64, only 13% of men and 15% of women ate 5 or more portions of fruit and vegetables per day. In fact, the 19-24 yr old men and women only consumed 1.3 and 1.8 portions, respectively, in comparison to the 50-64 yr olds where the figures were 3.6 and 3.8 portions. Even more worrying is the fact that in the 19-24 yr group, 45% and 27% of men and women, respectively, ate no fruit at all.

It has been estimated that increasing individual fruit and vegetable intake to at least 5-a-day could reduce coronary heart disease by 31% and ischaemic (the most common form of stroke) stroke by 19%. In addition, for stomach, oesophageal, lung and colorectal cancer, the estimated reductions could be 19%, 20%, 12% and 2%, respectively. However, due to hectic lifestyles, people prefer to have ready processed meals and pop a multivitamin rather than taking the trouble to buy and cook fresh food. **WE MUST REALISE that with many adults, in the short term, this situation will be hard to change due to constraints in time, attitude, education and finance.** The situation with children is more hopeful due to "5-a-day" campaigns underway focused in schools (see reference 94).

As a "normal" weight, healthy person in the 19-59 yr old group, is it necessary to take supplements and if so which ones? The answer will depend upon:

1. Your present diet
2. Your exposure to sunlight

1. Diet – If you are one of the 13% men and 15% women who eat at least 5 fruit or vegetables per day and have a well balanced diet then you may only require vitamin D (see 2. below). There is, however, as discussed in Chapter 7, no guarantee that your "well balanced" diet will contain all your daily requirements of vitamins/minerals due to loss of nutrients during food processing with the use of pesticides or poor storage and over cooking.

2. Exposure to sunlight – It is very difficult to obtain adequate requirements of vitamin D from the diet alone as exposure to sunlight is required for the body to make this vitamin. Indeed, it has been shown that of middle aged British adults, 60% are vitamin D deficient and this is particularly a problem during spring and winter when it may reach 90% (see reference 95).

In addition, you are likely to be very deficient in vitamin D if you are:

      a. Asian, Afro-Caribbean or Middle East in origin with very dark skin.

      b. Cover the skin through religious or health reasons.

      c. Rarely go outside the house (disabled or elderly).

      d. Do not eat much meat, oily fish or dairy products.

      e. Live in Scotland, Wales or other regions of the UK with little sunshine especially in the poor "summers" of 2007 and 2008.

Exposure of face, legs, arms etc to the sun for 10-15 minutes per day, 2-3 times per week without sunscreen (but with no burning), is recommended so the skin can make sufficient quantities of vitamin D_3 (the most beneficial kind). The body cannot over-produce vitamin D following excessive sun exposure. In addition, vitamin D produced can be stored so that intermittent sun exposure is fine.

In the UK, some foods, such as oily fish, naturally contain vitamin D while others have vitamins/minerals added (fortified). For example, margarine and reduced fat spreads have vitamin D added by law. The amount added, however, is only sufficient to match the levels found naturally in butter and **will not provide the shortfall arising from lack of exposure to the sun**. In addition, many breakfast cereals are also fortified with vitamins D and generally provide about 13% of adult vitamin D daily intake.

Despite this fortification, vitamin D deficiency in the UK is rife and the case for taking vitamin D supplements is extremely strong for the normal population as well as for the special groups of people identified below.

WHY HAVE I FOCUSED ON VITAMIN D SUPPLEMENTATION? Much recent research indicates that adequate intake of vitamin D helps to protect against:

        a. Cancers, including breast, prostate and colon

        b. Diabetes

        c. Problems with thinning of the bones (osteoporosis) resulting in falls and fractures in older, especially menopausal, females (see "Menopausal Women" and "People Over 50-60 yr" groups, below)

What other supplements are regularly taken by this group of 19-59 year old healthy people? These include:

a. Cod liver oil
b. Multivitamins
c. The antioxidant vitamins – A, C, E and selenium
d. Vitamin B
e. Calcium
f. Glucosamine

a. COD LIVER OIL OR FISH OILS for Omega-3 Fatty Acids. Many people take fish oil capsules regularly (1000 mg per day) to maintain and improve joint flexibility and relieve arthritic pain. In addition, fish oils may have many other benefits such as reducing the risk of heart disease, strokes and cancer and maintaining a healthy brain. Again, unfortunately, scientific opinion differs as to the benefits of taking fish oils although the weight of evidence does seem favorable (see reference 96). Taking omega-3 fish oils, which are present naturally in sardines, mackerel, herrings and salmon, in capsules is harmless and can therefore be recommended. Alternatively, eat 2 to 4 portions of oily fish per week such as tinned or fresh mackerel, salmon, trout, herrings, pilchards, kippers, anchovies, tuna (no more than 2 tuna steaks per week) and sardines, all of which contain natural omega-3 oils. Unfortunately, dioxins and mercury are pollutants that may be present at high levels in some oily fish such as shark, marlin, swordfish and types of fresh tuna and should be avoided by pregnant women (see reference 97). **Cod liver oil should be avoided by pregnant women and elderly people as it contains high vitamin A levels (see below). Also, see Chapter 7, Table 3, for correct sources of omega-3 fatty acids.**

b. MULTIVITAMINS are taken by large numbers of people in the belief that they will prevent heart disease, cancer and maintain general health and well-being. For normal people with balanced diets, including 5-a-day fruit or vegetables, there is very little evidence that multivitamins are beneficial in preventing disease. Thus, in 2006, the National Institute of Health (USA) concluded that there is insufficient evidence "to recommend either for or against the use of Multivitamin/Mineral Supplements to prevent chronic disease" (see reference 98). Unfortunately, few studies of multivitamins have been made although some reduction in cancer incidence has been reported (see references 99, 100). However, for many groups of people, including the over 50-60s, the obese, heavy drinkers and smokers (see below) with poor diets, multivitamins will probably be vital for filling gaps in their nutrition. **Most important is the fact that daily multivitamins appear to be safe as long as you check that they contain no more than the recommended daily allowance (=100% of RDA given in Tables 2, 3, Chapter 7)**

for the component vitamins and minerals and ONLY TAKE ONE PER DAY. The following Table 1 will allow you to confirm that your choice of multivitamin does not contain higher than recommended levels of supplements. It also indicates which supplements have been identified by the Foods Standards Agency (see reference 101) as causing side effects in excessive doses above the SUL (Safe Upper Limits as given in Tables 2, 3, Chapter 7).

Table 1. ADVICE TO CONSUMERS AND MANUFACTURERS ON UPPER THRESHOLD LEVELS OF SUPPLEMENTS*

Nutrient ↓	Threshold triggering advice	Advice of possible side effects
Calcium	More than 1500 mg	This amount of Calcium may cause mild stomach upset in sensitive people.
Iron	More than 20 mg	This amount of Iron may cause mild stomach upset in sensitive people.
Magnesium	More than 400 mg	This amount of Magnesium may cause mild stomach upset in sensitive people.
Manganese	More than 0.5 mg	Long term intake of this amount of Manganese may lead to muscle pain and fatigue.
Nickel	All nickel-containing products	Nickel may cause a skin rash in sensitive people.
Phosphorus	More than 250 mg	This amount of Phosphorus may cause mild stomach upsets in sensitive individuals".
Vitamin A (retinol, beta carotene)	More than 7 mg	Beta carotene may increase the risk of lung cancer in heavy smokers.
Vitamin B3 (niacin= nicotinic acid or nicotinamide)	More than 20 mg	Better as Nicotinamide form in supplement. If Nicotinic acid is used then this amount may cause skin flushes in sensitive people.
Vitamin B6	More than 10 mg	Long term intakes of this amount of vitamin B6 may lead to mild tingling and numbness. However, safe levels up to 100 mg have been advocated by many medical experts since excess is readily excreted from the body. Do not use high dosage without medical consultation.
Vitamin C	More than 1000 mg	This amount of Vitamin C may cause mild stomach upset in sensitive people.
Zinc	More than 25 mg	Long term intake of this amount of Zinc may lead to anaemia.

* See reference 101

The percentage RDA (recommended daily allowance) for each component is written on the multivitamin label. There are large numbers of different makes of multivitamins, for example, for children, the over 50s or pregnant women, so make sure you use the appropriate one and avoid excess of vitamin A or beta carotene (no more than 0.6-0.7 mg = 600-700 micrograms = 1998-2331 IU). BEWARE, AS OVER 50% OF MULTIVITAMINS MAY CONTAIN EXCESS VITAMIN A. A US study in 2000 of over 4500 female doctors showed that about 50% took a multivitamin-mineral supplement which is reassuring!

c. THE ANTIOXIDANT VITAMINS include A, C, E and selenium and are taken every day by millions of people in the UK, either in multivitamins or separately at higher doses. These antioxidants have been widely promoted as preventing many diseases such as cancer, heart problems and strokes as well as slowing down the aging process and halting Alzheimer's. This hype was based on the fact that antioxidants neutralise harmful oxygen radicals produced in the body as a result of many cellular activities associated with the utilisation of the oxygen that we breathe. These oxygen radicals then not only kill cells but also attack the DNA and cause mutations leading to aging, cancer and other diseases. **Many people became hooked on vitamin C in the 1970s as a result of:**

1. **Professor Linus Pauling**, a famous, 20th century, double Nobel Prize winning scientist, who advocated taking mega-doses (10-12 g daily!) of vitamin C for the prevention of the common cold, cardiovascular and other diseases (see reference 102).

2. **Media hype** of the benefits of antioxidants resulting from research publications on, for example, fruit flies and mice in which scientists engineered animals producing extra amounts of antioxidants in their bodies. The flies lived as much as 30% longer and the mice nearly 20% longer than animals producing normal levels of antioxidants (see references 103, 104). Thus in theory, we could all live beyond 100 yr old!

However, in the last few years, a number of high profile scientific reviews and organisations have questioned the effectiveness of antioxidant supplements in preventing disease. For example, the British Heart Foundation, (2002), the American Heart Association (2003), and the Foods Standards Agency (2003) have all stated that there is insufficient evidence to recommend taking antioxidants for the prevention or treatment of cancer or cardiovascular disease and advised against their use. A few reviews, including the Cochrane Review (2008) on antioxidants, have even indicated that high doses of antioxidants may be harmful (see reference 105). Needless to say, the media went wild and their headlines irresponsibly shouted out loud that all vitamins were dangerous! Thus, statements such as "Vitamin pill danger", "Vitamins could shorten lifespan" and "Vitamin tablets may do more harm than good" were splashed around everywhere. The end result is that the poor old public are totally confused as to whether taking vitamins is beneficial or harmful to health.

THE TRUTH OF THE MATTER IS THAT:

1. The majority of vitamins (including A, C, E and selenium) are safe provided that the recommended SULs (Safe Upper Limits) are not exceeded (see reference 101). These SULs are given in Tables 2 and 3 of Chapter 7. The reports of harmful effects are worth noting **but most negative reports are reviews** rather than original trials. Thus, the Cochrane Review (see reference 105) added together and then analysed the results of 67 previous clinical trials most of which used different doses and combinations of supplements as well as variable time scales and both healthy and sick patients. **Overall there was little evidence of increased risk of death from taking beta carotene or vitamins A, C, E or selenium** (see, however, "cigarette smokers", page 177 below). However, when the analytical technique was changed and the different antioxidants looked at separately there was a slight significant increase in risk of death with beta carotene (16% increase) and vitamins A (7%) and E (4%) but no increases for vitamin C or selenium. This is all very confusing and the techniques used unsatisfactory with the authors themselves concluding that further research was required.

2. Only you can decide whether you belong to the normal weight, healthy group of people eating at least 5-a-day fruit or vegetables and therefore do or do not require any antioxidant supplements.

3. Most healthy people in the 19-59 age group can obtain any additional antioxidant requirements from a one per day good multivitamin tablet.

4. If you decide to take higher levels of individual antioxidant   supplements (rarely recommended as evidence is mounting as to possible harmful effects) then it would be wise NOT to take a multivitamin as well and to limit yourself to:

   - Beta carotene/vitamin A - better not to supplement at all, especially smokers, pregnant women and the elderly

   - Vitamin C – no more than 250-500 mg/day

   - Vitamin E – no more than 200 IU (134mg) per day

   - Selenium – no more than 350-400 µg per day

5. Whatever you do, avoid advice from websites and magazines which are sponsored or linked to supplement manufacturers, otherwise you will end up spending a fortune on supplements that are unnecessary.

d. VITAMIN B SUPPLEMENTATION The need for vitamin B supplements by the healthy 19-59 yr olds is the subject of debate. Vitamin B is, however, recommended for many other groups of people including pregnant women, the elderly, drinkers, smokers and diabetics (see below).

There is some evidence for vitamin deficiency in healthy adults. For example, it was reported in 2000 that low levels of blood vitamin B-12 are present not only in 17% of the elderly (over 65 yr old) but also in a similar level of 26-64 yr old adults (see reference 106). In addition, about 3 million people in the UK take 100-200mg of vitamin B-6 daily for PMS (pre-menstrual stress), morning sickness or stress. Experimental evidence that high-dosage B6 alleviates this problem is disputed so maybe the effect produced is psychological (the placebo effect). The **patient's belief** that vitamin B-6 will improve their condition may bring about changes in body chemistry triggering the reduction in symptoms obtained.

There is also evidence that the B vitamins (folic acid = vitamin B-9, as well as B-6 and B-12), may help to break down an amino acid in the blood called homocysteine. High homocysteine levels have been linked to heart disease and strokes by promoting the formation of fatty deposits in the arteries and blood clot formation. Much research has been undertaken to prove the role of homocysteine in cardiovascular disease. To date, although heart patients have raised levels of homocysteine, its exact role in heart disease is unknown (see, however, reference 107). Lowering homocysteine by increasing folic acid (B-9), B-6 and B-12 intakes have been advocated to reduce the risk of heart disease.

Increased vitamin B intake can be obtained directly from the diet with 5-a-day fruit and vegetables (see Table 2, Chapter 7) and from vitamin fortified breakfast cereals and bread. Again, if you avoid breakfast cereals or bread and fail to eat sufficient fruit and vegetables then a vitamin supplement will be required. A multivitamin should contain at least 400 micrograms of folic acid but optimal levels of B-6 and B-12 have not been determined. Daily doses of 12.5 mg for B-6 and 500 micrograms for B-12 are safe as long as they do not interact with other drugs being taken. Each of these B vitamins, but particularly folic acid, may contribute to reducing homocysteine so do not worry if your multivitamin does not contain all three.

e. CALCIUM SUPPLEMENTATION may be required if you avoid dairy produce due to lactose intolerance or adopt a vegan lifestyle. For normal people, more than 70% of calcium is taken up from dairy produce although fortified foods such as bread and some cereals are also important sources. All flour in the UK is fortified with calcium except wholemeal which naturally contains 380mg calcium per kilogram. As a rough guide, you need 800-1500 mg of calcium per day and 3 cups of milk (or yoghurt) will provide about 900 mg. See Table 3 in Chapter 7 for other food sources of calcium.

Calcium supplements are one of the most popular mineral supplements in the USA and UK.

Again, it is for you to judge whether you have enough dairy produce and/or fortified food each day to obtain the necessary 800-1500 mg of calcium. Special groups of people who are more likely to require calcium supplements are young children (800 mg) to ensure they have strong bones as well as pregnant and nursing mothers (1200-1500 mg), menopausal women and elderly people (1500 mg). See details for some of these groups below and consult with your doctor about supplementation.

If you do decide to take a calcium supplement then be aware that calcium may inhibit the absorption of iron. Check to make sure that your multivitamin does not contain both iron and calcium. In addition, fibre in food may bind to calcium and inhibit uptake so vegans/vegetarians beware. It is therefore recommended that calcium pills are taken 1-2 hr after a meal and no more than 500 mg should be taken each time. Make sure that you have sufficient vitamin D (see above) which will aid in the absorption of calcium.

f. GLUCOSAMINE is taken by people from middle age onwards for the reduction of joint pain and inflammation, often associated with osteoarthritis, and to assist with joint mobility. Over 2 million people in the UK suffer from osteoarthritis with the average age of onset about 45 years old. The dose usually recommended orally is 1500 mg per day and should be taken for 6-8 weeks to see if symptoms improve. Glucosamine is not a registered medicine in the UK and therefore is a supplement which may or may not provide relief. Generally, glucosamine is safe to take long-term except for people with allergies to shellfish. Sometimes glucosamine is taken with chondroitin sulphate as this combination may provide further benefit for people with osteoarthritis (see reference 108). A recent study concluded, however, that glucosamine sulphate (1500 mg daily) was ineffective for treating hip osteoarthritis (see reference 109). A controversy thus exists so the best thing to do is to try glucosamine if you suffer from osteoarthritis and see if your symptoms improve. Also, note the warning in Table 3, Chapter 7, about not taking glucosamine **sulphate** but glucosamine **hydrochloride** instead, if you have high blood pressure.

SUMMARY RECOMMENDATION FOR "NORMAL" HEALTHY PEOPLE 19-59 YEARS OLD

+++ vitamin D

BUT if you do not eat at least 5 fruit or vegetable portions per day (over 80% of this group) and also do not have sufficient dairy produce in your diet then you may require supplementation with one or more of the following:

+++ multivitamin (preferably without vitamin A)

+++ vitamin D and calcium

++   omega-3 fish oil (not cod liver oil)

++   glucosamine for osteoarthritis sufferers usually over 40 years old

++   vitamin B from multivitamin (see above) or from a separate supplement to get higher levels of B-6 and B-12

All daily

NB: If you are taking any medicines then check with your medical advisor that these will not interact with the vitamin pills

ii. PREGNANT WOMEN Women intending to conceive or who are pregnant are recommended to take 400 micrograms of **folic acid (vitamin B9)** per day as a supplement to reduce the chances of spina bifida. If a spina bifida baby was born previously, this should be increased to 5mg of folic acid. More recently, the Department of Health has also advised pregnant and breast-feeding women to take a 10 microgram per day **vitamin D** supplement to avoid problems with skeletal development (rickets). This is especially important in the winter when vitamin D cannot be made by the body due to lack of exposure to the sun. Iron supplements are not recommended by the UK Food Standards Agency unless the woman is anaemic. Pregnant women should be tested for anaemia routinely. Many women take a multivitamin-mineral supplement prior to and during pregnancy. This is beneficial for those foolish enough to smoke and drink whilst pregnant but **make sure that such multivitamins do not contain vitamin A which can cause foetal malformations.** Many multivitamins carry no warning over the dangers of vitamin A to the baby. Avoid foods and supplements like liver, pate and fish oils (eg. cod liver oil) with high levels of vitamin A (**http://www.eatwell.gov.uk**). Maternal omega-3 fish oil supplementation during pregnancy has also been shown to be safe for the foetus and infant, and may have beneficial effects on the child's eye and hand coordination, although more evidence is required before strong recommendation can be made. Tinned or fresh mackerel, salmon, trout, herring, kippers, pilchards, anchovies, fresh tuna (no more than one 6 oz tuna steak per week) and sardines naturally contain beneficial omega-3 oils. Avoid eating shark, swordfish and marlin steaks which can be high in mercury (see reference 97).

SUMMARY RECOMMENDATION

+++   folic acid
+++   vitamin D (usually D3 recommended)
++   omega-3 fish oils, 1000 mg per day, if intolerant of 2-4 portions of oily fish each week

All daily

iii. BREAST FEEDING WOMEN like pregnant women should boost their intake of **vitamin D.** In addition, if the pregnant or nursing mother does not have a diet high in calcium, since she may avoid dairy products through allergy etc, then a **calcium supplement** may be required and she should consult with her GP. Multivitamins may be recommended, but those made especially for nursing mothers should be used.

SUMMARY RECOMMENDATION

+++   vitamin D
++   multivitamin
+   calcium

All daily

iv. BABIES AND INFANTS less than 6 months old and fed on breast milk or formula milk should not need supplements. If breast-fed then after 6 months **vitamin A, C and D supplements** (as liquid drops) may be required but only under direction of a health visitor/doctor. These can be continued until 5 yr old if the child eats poorly or is not exposed to the sun for short times.

SUMMARY RECOMMENDATION

+   vitamins A, C and D (liquid drops)

All daily

v. SCHOOL CHILDREN may have poor diets with less than half surveyed eating the 5 a day fruit and vegetables required. Approximately, 20% of 4-18 year olds eat no fruit at all (see reference 110). In addition, about 20% of UK teenagers are obese with numbers having tripled since 1980. Up to 10% of teenage girls may also be vegetarians or on special diets. It is no wonder that teenagers are reported to have low intakes of vitamin A, D and riboflavin (vitamin B2) as well as the minerals, calcium, zinc, iron and magnesium. Lectures on healthy eating are often ignored. It has been shown that **taking a multivitamin supplement** is highly beneficial for teens and associated with healthier lifestyles (see reference 111). Since over 70% of teenage girls may also be vitamin D deficient (see reference 112), supplementation may be highly beneficial. Multivitamins for teens contain 2.5-5 micrograms (100-200 IU) of vitamin D.

SUMMARY RECOMMENDATION

+++   multivitamin

++   vitamin D daily but only if multivitamin not taken daily

vi. WOMEN WITH HEAVY PERIODS are particularly prone to **iron deficiency anaemia** due to excessive loss of blood and will benefit from iron supplementation under supervision. Teenage girls with diets rich in sugar, snacks and crisps, which interfere with iron uptake, may also be in need of additional iron. Eating vitamin C–rich foods such as fruit, juices and vegetables (see Table 2, Chapter 7) will aid in iron absorption. Women using oral contraceptives may have reduced bleeding during periods and are less likely to require iron supplements. Vitamin D is recommended (400 IU =10 micrograms daily) during the winter months or if not exposed to sunlight for about 15 min twice per week without sunscreen greater than factor 8.

SUMMARY RECOMMENDATION

++   iron

++   vitamin D

Both daily

vii. MENOPAUSAL AND POST-MENOPAUSAL WOMEN

Recommending supplements for these groups of women is controversial. Neither the Foods Standards Agency nor the British Nutrition Foundation recommends specific supplementation for women at these stages, although they emphasise the importance of a balanced diet. Women on iron supplements can stop using these when menstrual bleeding reduces during the menopause. For women not on Hormone Replacement Therapy (HRT), a whole range of supplements have been recommended to alleviate menopausal symptoms and bone loss resulting from osteoporosis or bone thinning and resulting in increased fractures. These supplements include vitamins A, B, C, D, E and K, as well as the minerals, calcium and magnesium, and plant/herb extracts containing phytoestrogens such as dong quai, black cohosh, red clover and soya. Evidence is limited or controversial as to the beneficial effects of using most of these. The case, however, for the use of calcium and vitamin D supplements is gradually being accepted as is the need for a revision upwards of the safe upper limits in the use of vitamin D (see reference 113). Old upper safety limits for vitamin D were originally set over 30 years ago to prevent rickets. **Evidence now indicates that supplementation with 700-800 IU (17.5-20 microgram) vitamin D results in fewer fractures, with or without a calcium supplement.** Cod liver oil contains not only high levels of vitamin D but also vitamin A which can be toxic so it is better to use a pure vitamin D supplement. Vitamin E and black cohosh may also reduce hot flushes, but beware of using any herbs with the Pill or HRT.

SUMMARY RECOMMENDATION

+++   vitamin D
+   calcium

Both daily

viii. PEOPLE OVER 50-60 YR OLD   must avoid at all costs:

"THE DOWNWARD SPIRAL OF AGING"

This process results from older people:

1. Eating less or buying lower quality food because of reduced incomes

2. Eating less food due to dental problems and inability to chew effectively

3. Having a reduced efficiency for digestion and absorption of food by the gut which may be related to loss of acid production in the stomach

4. Living alone due to loss of partner or divorce and a reduced incentive to prepare regular and well balanced meals

5. Confined indoors, away from sunlight, due to illness or social isolation, resulting in vitamin deficiency

6. Commonly taking medications such as antibiotics that may interfere with vitamin and mineral absorption

7. Suffering malnutrition as a result of 1-6 (above) and losing weight, strength and energy for exercise

8. Having little exercise which accelerates loss of muscle and bone mass (see, "Sarcopenia" and "Osteoporosis" Chapter 11, pages 217-220), reduced strength and results in frailty, more frequent falls, fractures and infections

9. Loss of independence

10. Admission into Care Home or Hospital

Figure 1. Showing components of the "Downward Spiral of Aging"

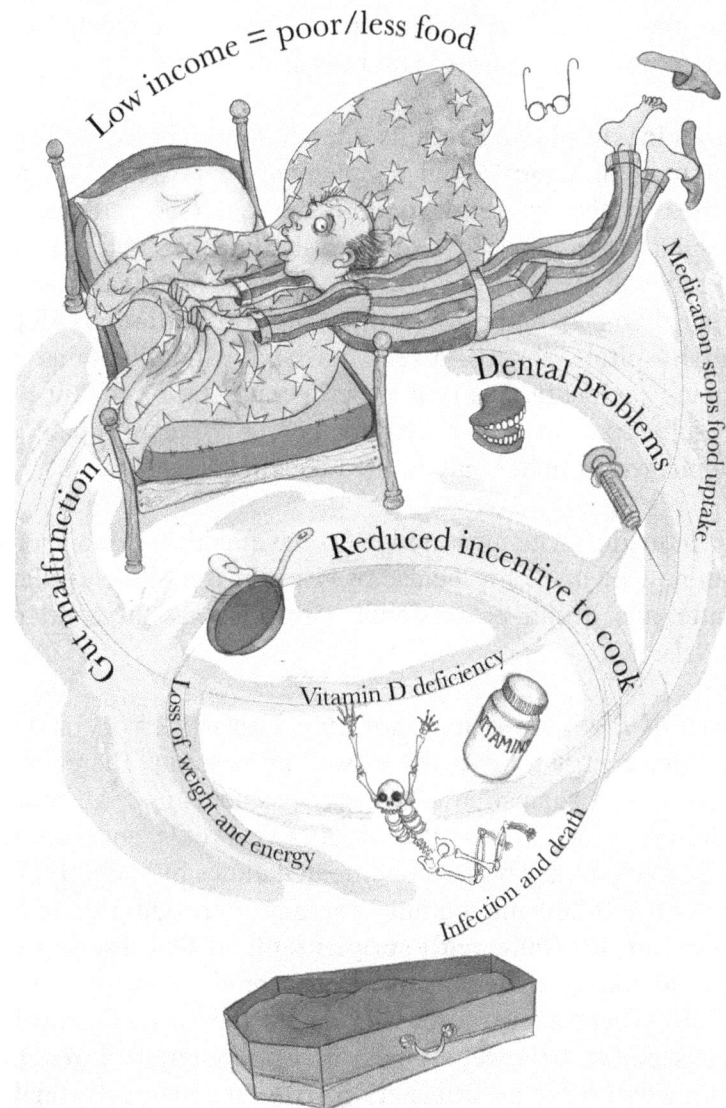

The aging process is thus accelerated by a downward spiral of malnutrition, weakness, frailty, reduced immune efficiency and infection. These processes may be accelerated both in care homes and hospitals. Elderly people are therefore prime candidates for vitamin supplementation.

Even so, supplement recommendation for elderly people is a controversial subject since so many older people are taking medicines, which may interact with nutrient/supplement absorption. There are also few studies of the effects of supplementation in the older person. All the recommended daily allowances (RDAs) of vitamins and minerals in Tables 2 and 3 in Chapter 7 have been derived from research with people in the 19-59 age group. Obviously, if an elderly relative is involved, it is better to supervise an improved diet with 5-a-day fruit and vegetables and well balanced meals (see Chapters 1 and 7), as vitamins are more easily absorbed naturally from food.

A **multivitamin supplement** seems the obvious choice and yet some trials of the beneficial effects of multivitamin supplements have failed to detect any reduction in infection rates in elderly people over 65 yr old (see reference 114). Possibly, these negative results occurred because some of the vitamins and minerals in the multivitamin pills interfered with the absorption of each other. Also, these trials tended to **use healthy, older people living at home** rather than more **nutritionally-deprived people in care homes and hospitals**. Indeed, a few trials with multivitamins have recorded reduced infection rates in institutionalized older people (see reference 115). Perhaps these contrary results confirm that providing people have adequate diets then at any age vitamin supplementation has only limited benefits.

Trials with individual vitamins, however, have achieved more promising results. Thus, the case can now be made for the use of **vitamin B and D supplements in older people** but only after the health professional confirms that these do not interfere with any medication taken.

A **deficiency of B vitamins** may not only impair memory and alertness but can also result in reduced energy for exercise as well as anaemia. There are also indications that B vitamins can protect against strokes, heart problems and Alzheimer's disease. **Vitamin B12 deficiency** occurs in 10-15% of 60+ year olds and can result in anaemia and dementia-like symptoms which can be treated either by monthly injections of 1 mg or by supplements of 100-200 micrograms per day, depending on the extent of deficiency. Recently, **vitamin B9 (folic acid) supplements of 800 micrograms per day** have also been shown to improve the memories and brain power of 50 to 70 year olds (see reference 116). There is also discussion about the **role of vitamin B6** in dementia and mental processes. **On balance, vitamin B supplementation would seem worthwhile in elderly people assuming no interaction with any drugs prescribed.** In the USA, there has been fortification of cereals with folic acid for the last 10 years.

There is some controversy regarding **supplementation with Vitamin D** but in people, such as the elderly deprived of sunlight, **a dose of 700-800 IU (17.5-20 micrograms) per day** is recommended to reduce falls and fractures (see, previous section, "menopausal and post-menopausal women"). The use of vitamin D supplements may also increase life expectancy significantly (see reference 117). In addition, since vitamin D and calcium work together in the body, it is recommended **to take a calcium supplement of not more than 1500 mg per day** to slow down bone loss in the elderly. Again, controversy exists over the use of these supplements so consult your doctor first.

Studies have also discussed the **benefits of taking vitamins C and E as well as selenium and zinc**. Again, there is controversy since there are reports that using C, E and selenium might increase the incidence of certain cancers. In contrast, there is evidence for a protective role with vitamins C and E against Alzheimer's disease but only at much higher doses than present in multivitamins. Thus, 500 mg of vitamin C and 400 IU vitamin E would be required and there is evidence that vitamin E at this level could be harmful. Thus, improving the diet rather than overdosing on vitamins C and E would be optimal. Selenium is an important antioxidant, levels of which have been declining in the UK diet with the institutionalised elderly at the greatest risk of deficiency. A **supplement of 50 micrograms per day** can be taken with no side effects but it is better to confirm deficiency with a blood test first. The case for **supplementing with zinc (10mg per day) is strongest** for elderly people to boost their immune system and prevent infections such as pneumonia.

Many elderly people also take **fish oil capsules regularly (1000 mg per day)** to maintain and improve joint flexibility and relieve arthritic pain. In addition, fish oils may have many other benefits such as reducing the risk of heart disease, strokes and cancer. Again, unfortunately, scientific opinion differs as to the benefits of taking fish oils although the weight of evidence does seem favorable. In addition, recent research has also shown that omega-3 fish oils can help combat Alzheimer's disease but only in certain people **without a gene predisposing them to developing Alzheimer's** (see reference 118). Taking omega-3 fish oils, which are present naturally in sardines, mackerel, herrings and salmon, is harmless and is therefore recommended. Do buy a good quality omega-3 free of dioxin and mercury.

The Food Standards Agency (www.**eatwell.gov.uk**) recommends that elderly people avoid fish liver oils, such as **COD LIVER OIL** supplements, as they contain high quantities of vitamin A which can result in loss of bone density, osteoporosis and increase in bone fractures. Cod liver oil supplements for elderly people have recently been recommended by a TV doctor who should know better

Finally, many elderly people also take **glucosamine sulphate** supplements for osteoarthritis which affects the joints. This supplement may reduce joint pain and inflammation and assist with joint mobility. The dose usually recommended orally is 1500 mg per day and it should be taken for 6-8 weeks to see if symptoms improve. Glucosamine is not a registered medicine in the UK and therefore is a supplement which may or may not provide relief. Generally, glucosamine is safe to take long-term except for people with allergies to shellfish. Sometimes glucosamine is taken with chondroitin sulphate as this combination may provide further benefit for people with osteoarthritis (see reference 108). A recent study (see reference 109) concluded, however, that glucosamine sulphate (1500 mg daily) was ineffective for treating hip osteoarthritis. A controversy thus exists so that the best thing to do is to try glucosamine if you suffer from osteoarthritis and see if your symptoms improve. Check Table 3, Chapter 7, for use of glucosamine hydrochloride instead of sulphate in cases of high blood pressure.

SUMMARY RECOMMENDATION

> **NB: If you are taking any medicines then check with your medical advisor that these will not interact with the vitamin pills**

+++   multivitamin for elderly in care/hospital (preferably without vitamin A)

+++   vitamin D* and calcium**

++   omega-3 fish oil (not cod liver oil)

++   glucosamine for osteoarthritis sufferers

++   vitamin B* from multivitamin (above) but if very deficient in vitamin B 12 then 1 mg per month of B 12 injected or a 100-200 microgram tablet daily dissolved under the tongue

All the above daily

*NB: Both vitamins B and D may be present in the multivitamin (as in the Boots multivitamin for the over 50s) in which case these may not have to be taken again separately. If levels of vitamins B and D are very low in the multivitamin, it may be necessary to take these separately. If the multivitamin contains iron, this may compete with calcium for absorption by the gut, in which case take your calcium supplement (with food but not with caffeine drinks) some hours after the multivitamin.

**There is some discussion as to whether calcium supplements can cause hardening of the arteries and heart attacks/strokes but further research is needed. In the meantime, if over 70 yr old, eat more high calcium-rich foods and reduce calcium supplements (for reassurance see reference 119). This study looked at over 36,000, 50-79 yr old women and found no adverse effects of calcium supplements.

ix. PEOPLE IN HOSPITAL/CARE HOMES. These include sick people with long stays in hospital and disabled or others, such as Alzheimer's patients, in care. This group includes elderly people (see above) who are likely to be malnourished and would benefit from a multivitamin and, if confined indoors, also vitamin D. To avoid interactions with any medication, check with a health professional before taking supplements.

SUMMARY RECOMMENDATION

+++   multivitamin (without vitamin A if possible)
+++   vitamin D

Both daily

x. CIGARETTE SMOKERS are damaging the DNA and organs throughout their bodies, including the lungs, gut and heart, due to the oxidative stress resulting from the chemicals in cigarette smoke. This will often lead to cancer, cardiovascular disease and accelerated aging. Smoking reduces levels of antioxidants such as vitamins C and E which can defend the body against the ravages of smoking (see reference 120). In addition, it has been shown that levels of the B vitamins, such as B6, B9 and B12, are also lower in smokers.

RECENT RESEARCH HAS SHOWN THAT SMOKING INCREASES THE RISK OF DEMENTIA AND ALZHEIMER'S DISEASE

A vitamin C supplement of 1000 mg per day has been reported to significantly reduce the loss of vitamin E caused by smoking. It is also better to take a separate vitamin B supplement since multivitamins often contain vitamin A.

DO NOT TAKE VITAMIN A OR VITAMIN E SUPPLEMENTS IF YOU SMOKE AS THESE MAY INCREASE THE INCIDENCE OF LUNG CANCER

SUMMARY RECOMMENDATION

+++   vitamin C
++   vitamin B
++   vitamin D

All daily

xi. DRINKERS are likely to be to be suffering from multiple vitamin deficiencies. This is true not only for alcoholics but also for binge drinkers at the weekend and for people drinking regularly throughout the week with friends or during work. This vitamin deficiency results from both a poor diet, which drinkers often have, and from alcohol inhibiting the uptake of vitamins and increasing their breakdown in the stomach. **Vitamins particularly affected are B1 (thiamine), B2 (riboflavin), B6 (pyridoxine), B9 (folic acid) and vitamin C.** The extent of any deficiency will depend upon the amount and regularity of drinking as well as upon the normal intake of vitamins in the diet. In addition, vitamins A, D and E as well as vital minerals such as calcium, zinc, iron and magnesium may also be deficient in alcoholics. The results of these alcohol-induced deficiencies will vary from one person to another but can have serious consequences. Thus, folic acid deficiency has been reported to be linked to anaemia, cancer of the colon, Alzheimer's and foetal damage, while **long-term thiamine (B1) deficiency can result in severe brain damage and dementia.**

> **RECENT WORK HAS SHOWN THAT WHEN HEAVY DRINKING IS ASSOCIATED WITH SMOKING THEN THE AGE OF ONSET OF ALZHEIMER'S DISEASE CAN BE 6-7 YEARS EARLIER**
> (see reference 121)

The research showed:

- Heavy drinkers developed Alzheimer's 4.8 years earlier than non-drinkers or light drinkers.

- Heavy smokers developed Alzheimer's 2.3 years earlier than non-smokers or light smokers.

- Those people who drank and smoked heavily but also had the APOE4 gene, which increases the risk of Alzheimer's, developed the disease 8.5 years earlier than those without the three risk factors.

> **HEAVY DRINKERS WERE DEFINED AS THOSE WHO HAD MORE THAN TWO DRINKS EVERY DAY, WHILE HEAVY SMOKERS HAD 20 OR MORE CIGARETTES PER DAY**

A TRUE AND SAD STORY

This involved my sister who died recently from Alzheimer's disease at the age of 66. She was an ex beauty queen, London fashion model and then a famous astrologer. She wrote for many of the daily and weekend national newspapers, including the Sunday Mirror, Daily Express and Daily Star, as well as appearing regularly on Living TV. Unfortunately, her astrology writing meant that for many years she was confined for months on end in her study trying to meet deadlines for her 12 monthly astrology guides published each year. In addition, like many people, she had marital problems, and the stress of these and her need to meet tight deadlines resulted in more and more excessive smoking and drinking. Eventually, I noticed changes in her appearance and eyesight both of which gradually degenerated. Like the rest of her family, however, I had no idea as to the level of her drinking until large numbers of empty vodka bottles were found in her study. Her behaviour became more and more eccentric and her short-term memory practically non-existent. Eventually her appearance, memory and behaviour necessitated medical scrutiny and resulted in the diagnosis of Alzheimer's disease. This was followed by her institutionalization and, finally, her death in just a few years. Her decline was no doubt hastened by a poor diet, including excessive amounts of cheese, which would have raised her cholesterol levels to possibly contribute to her early onset of dementia. Thus, I lost a beautiful and dearly beloved sister to excessive stress, drinking and smoking coupled to a poor diet – factors that often go hand-in-hand.

DOES ANY OF THIS SOUND FAMILIAR TO YOU?

SUMMARY RECOMMENDATION

It is difficult to be precise in making recommendations for drinkers as a lot will depend upon the amount drunk and how frequently. Alcoholics may need emergency treatment and institutionalizing with daily injection of high dose vitamins. Regular and binge drinkers would do well to take:

+++   a multivitamin tablet daily

+++   vitamin B complex 100-300 mg daily, the dose taken depending upon both the amount drunk daily and the nutritional value of the diet

+++   vitamin C by eating more fruit but also by at least a 500 mg tablet daily

xii. DIABETICS There are about 2 million diagnosed diabetic adults in England, with numbers rising at an alarming rate. With a body mass index (BMI) in excess of 30 there is as much as a ten-fold increase in risk of becoming diabetic. There are also ethnic groups at particular risk of developing diabetes including Afro-Caribbeans and Asians. **Most importantly, recent research indicates that levels of specific vitamins can be linked to both the risk of developing diabetes as well as preventing the complications resulting in heart disease, strokes, blindness, kidney and nerve damage.** Thus, **low levels of vitamin D**, due to low intake or lack of exposure to the sun, may increase the risk of developing diabetes. This might explain why dark-skinned people, who are less able to make their own vitamin D, are more prone to develop diabetes. In addition, low vitamin D levels in diabetics are correlated with complications such as cardiovascular disease (see review reference 122). Even more recently, research has shown that **diabetics have blood levels of vitamin B1 (thiamine) which are about 75% lower than in normal people**. Since thiamine is important in maintaining healthy blood vessels then this thiamine deficiency in diabetics may be linked to the many complications of diabetes (see reference 123).

SUMMARY RECOMMENDATION

+++ vitamin D, some people have a 33% reduced risk of diabetes if taking 800 IU (20 micrograms) vitamin D together with 1200 mg of calcium daily. Consult your doctor

+++ vitamin B1 (thiamine), supplementation of diabetic patients' diet with thiamine is on trial, but it is worthwhile taking a vitamin B supplement in a multivitamin until optimal levels have been determined

Both daily

xiii. PEOPLE WITH GUT PROBLEMS There are a range of conditions that can lead to the poor absorption (malabsorption) of nutrients, such as vitamins and minerals, from food. Thus, malabsorption can occur with **Crohn's disease, ulcerative colitis, inflammatory bowel syndrome, coeliac disease, food allergy/intolerance, gut infections and cancer**. Such diseases will have to be diagnosed and treated medically. In some of these conditions, vitamin supplementation is unnecessary as with allergic or intolerance reactions to food, for example, **coeliac disease** caused by sensitivity to the gluten protein present in cereals or with **lactose intolerance** to dairy products. Simply avoiding these foods may rectify the problem. With other conditions, including **Crohn's disease**, multiple vitamin and mineral deficiencies can occur. Thus, deficiencies in many vitamins including A, B1, B2, B6, folic acid, B12, E and K as well as the minerals, zinc, calcium and magnesium have been found (reviewed in reference 124). Likewise with **cancer of the gut, pancreas, liver or gallbladder,** there may be multiple impairment of the digestion and absorption of vitamins and minerals and other nutrients. Whether supplements are required and how to take them will depend upon **diagnosis of the type and severity of the disease.** In some cases, adjustments to the diet will be sufficient (eg. coeliac disease) while in others, supplements will need to be injected or given directly into the veins (cancer).

SUMMARY RECOMMENDATION

+++ multivitamin daily BUT depends on which disease and it's severity

Supplementation should be given under the direction of a health professional

xiv. OVERWEIGHT OR OBESE PEOPLE In the UK more than 50% of adults are overweight (BMI 25-30) and about 23% of these are obese (BMI over 30).

Many overweight people have poor diets rich in fatty and sugary foods and alcohol but low in fruit, vegetables and dairy products. In addition, they may struggle unsuccessfully with various diets such as the Atkins which are low in fruits and vegetables. The end result is that overweight people often have vitamin and mineral deficiencies but particularly vitamins B6 (pyridoxine), C, D and E, and if they are dieting they may lack minerals such as iron, calcium and zinc. Taking a multivitamin and mineral supplement is recommended regardless of whether dieting or not. Vitamin D deficiency has now been shown to be higher in obese people than in the normal population (see reference 125).

SUMMARY RECOMMENDATION

+++ a multivitamin tablet
+++ vitamin D (10 micrograms, 400IU)

Both daily

xv. VEGANS, VEGETARIANS AND PEOPLE ON DIETS are likely to be deficient in certain key vitamins and minerals. This group will include not only overweight people (see: "Overweight or Obese People", above) but also those on special diets such as vegans and vegetarians. Between 3% and 7% of the UK population are

vegetarians and these include vegans who avoid all food of animal origin. Sometimes, people adopting a vegetarian lifestyle may have mineral or vitamin deficiencies due to a lack of knowledge of the optimal foods to eat. Vegetarians may need supplements containing vitamins B12 and D as well as calcium, iron and zinc, all of which are present in meat and dairy produce. **Vitamin B12 is a particular need in vegetarians** since it is not present in plant tissues and deficiency may lead to anaemia and nerve damage. Yeast extracts and Marmite are sources of B12 as are some foods such as soya milk and breakfast cereals fortified with this vitamin (read the labels). **Vitamin D deficiency is widespread in the normal UK population but some vegetarians (especially vegans) will be even more deficient** since dietary sources of vitamin D are of animal origin, including liver, dairy produce and oily fish. Some dairy-free milks and margarines are fortified with vitamin D (but with very low levels) and free of harmful hydrogenated fats (trans fats). **Calcium, iron and zinc can all be obtained from the vegetarian diet.** Details of plant sources of these minerals are given in Table 3 of Chapter 7.

SUMMARY RECOMMENDATION

+++ a multivitamin tablet for dieters
+++ vitamin B12 for vegetarians with 100-200* microgram tablet dissolved under the tongue
+++ vitamin D (10 micrograms, 400IU)

All daily

* there is disagreement as to the exact dose of vitamin B12 required as a supplement.

xvi. PEOPLE WHO EXERCISE REGULARLY should not normally require any further vitamin and mineral supplementation in addition to those recommended for "Normal Healthy People 19-59 Years Old" (see p.155, above). During exercise, the body uses more oxygen which results in the formation of additional oxygen radicals that may damage the tissues. Research, however, seems to indicate that the body can compensate naturally for this additional oxidative stress by increased production of antioxidant enzymes without the need to take antioxidant supplements (see review reference 126). It is, however, important to emphasise that people taking regular exercise need to have a balanced diet to provide the necessary calories for energy production, protein for tissue repair and fruit and vegetables as sources of antioxidants. **With endurance athletes, such as regular marathon runners, tri-athletes, cyclists etc, there is, however, some evidence that antioxidant supplements may offer protection** against the very high levels (10-20 times resting state levels) of radicals generated by these sports. Thus, an **increased intake of vitamin E**

may be protective but precise levels are unknown although 100-200 IU per day has been recommended. In addition, since some athletes may restrict their intake of calories and certain food groups, they may have vitamin or mineral deficiencies. A **multivitamin-mineral supplement containing a range of B-vitamins** will ensure that energy production and muscle repair are optimal.

SUMMARY RECOMMENDATION

++ vitamin E may protect **endurance athletes** against oxidative stress

++ a multivitamin-mineral supplement for **endurance athletes** will ensure that performance is not inhibited by deficiencies

Both daily

FROM THE ABOVE, WE CAN ESTIMATE THAT ABOUT 45 MILLION PEOPLE FROM A POPULATION IN THE UK OF 61.4 MILLION BELONG TO GROUPS LIKELY TO BENEFIT FROM VITAMIN/MINERAL SUPPLEMENTS

TIPS ON BUYING VITAMINS AND MINERALS Deciding which make of vitamins/minerals to buy can be a difficult task with prices for apparently similar products being highly variable. In addition, supplements can be expensive and nobody wishes to spend more than necessary. Having decided, from reading the above and chapter 7, the type and strength of vitamins required then it is essential to be confident that the brand(s) chosen meets your requirements. Remember, the following points only need to be considered before your **first** purchase:

1. Read the labels on the bottle and check that the pills contain the appropriate vitamin/mineral dose required and are not out of date.

2. Also look for any **warnings of interactions with certain medicines given in the instructions in each packet** (see below, page 186).

3. When buying multivitamins, make sure that you purchase **the correct type** required i.e. for children, pregnant or nursing mothers, or people over 50 yr old etc.

4. With a multivitamin, double check that the RDA (recommended daily allowance) for vitamin A or beta-carotene **is not above 100%.**

5. Many vitamins are synthetic rather than "natural" or "organic" and there is "evidence" that **some natural vitamins**, such as vitamin E, are not only **absorbed more effectively in the gut but utilised better** by the body. Natural vitamin E will be labelled "d-alpha-tocopherol" and synthetic "dl-alpha-tocopherol".

6. **There is very little regulation regarding the production of supplements** and no guarantee that they contain the amount of vitamin/mineral written on the label. If you really need to check the quality of supplements then enquire in the shop and failing a satisfactory answer (probably) ask for a contact telephone number. A reputable manufacturer should be able to provide answers/proof of their quality control processes. In the UK, information about vitamins and supplements is available in Holland and Barrett and Boots stores from trained personnel who should help. In the USA, supplements can be checked out at **www.supplementquality.com/testing/Quality_seals.html**. Note that the European Commission has a Working Group considering setting maximum and minimum levels of vitamins and minerals in foodstuffs such as supplements (see reference 127).

FOR FUN WITH THE CHILDREN why not carry out a simple experiment. Vitamin and mineral pills not only contain the supplement required but also fillers, binders and coatings to stabilise and hold the pill together. **It is worthwhile checking if the pills taken dissolve in the gut to release their contents** for absorption by the body or whether they pass straight through the gut into the toilet. Simply place some vinegar in a heat-proof container and heat on a hotplate to 98° F = body temperature (take care with the hotplate). Put the test pill in the container, maintain the temperature and stir every few minutes without touching the pill. The pill should dissolve by 30-45 min unless it is labelled "enteric coated" or "slow release" which should be resistant to the acid in the stomach represented by the vinegar. If it dissolves too quickly then this is also of concern as the contents may be broken down and destroyed in the stomach.

TIPS ON TAKING VITAMIN/MINERAL SUPPLEMENTS

1. **To aid in their absorption, these should generally be taken with a meal or snack**. This is especially important with the fat-soluble vitamins such as vitamins A, D and E, beta carotene and coenzyme Q10. Make sure that the **food contains a little fat** (no, not a bacon buttie!) which will aid in the absorption of these latter vitamins. Excess of these fat-soluble vitamins are stored in the body and therefore do not exceed the correct dose.

2. **Other vitamins, such as B and C, dissolve in water** and will rapidly pass out of the body in the urine unless taken with food. Some vitamins, such as vitamin C, are sold as "enteric-coated" or "slow release" and will survive passage through the acid in the stomach into the small intestine for better absorption.

3. **Do not take your vitamins with hot drinks or drinks containing caffeine** which is present in tea, coffee, colas etc. Caffeine inhibits the absorption of some vitamins and minerals, such as iron, and stimulates the loss of others, such as calcium, from the body.

4. **Calcium may inhibit the absorption of iron** so do not take both at the same time. In addition, **fibre in food may bind to calcium** and inhibit uptake so vegans/vegetarians beware. Therefore, **take calcium pills 1-2 hr after a meal** and no more than 500mg should be taken each time.

5. Most people take vitamins as tablets or capsules, however, **there are liquid vitamins** for people who find pills difficult to swallow. Liquid vitamins tend to be expensive and could potentially lose more of their activity in the acid of the stomach than tablet forms, especially more than enteric-coated pills.

INTERACTIONS OF VITAMINS WITH MEDICINES

IF YOU HAVE A MEDICAL CONDITION IT IS MOST IMPORTANT TO CONSULT YOUR DOCTOR BEFORE TAKING SUPPLEMENTS

It is natural for sick people to take supplements in the hope of "strengthening" their immune systems and speeding recovery. Cancer patients, in particular, are amongst the highest users of supplements. There are **many accounts of the interactions of vitamins and minerals with medicines** with some of these scientifically proven while others are more theoretical and the basis of cautionary advice. For example:

1. There is much cautionary advice about cancer patients not taking high doses of antioxidants like vitamins A and E as these may not only interfere with the action of chemotherapeutic drugs but also stimulate cancer cell growth.

2. Folic acid (vitamin B-9) can interfere with some drugs used to treat epilepsy and inflammation.

3. Riboflavin (vitamin B-3) impairs the activity of some (streptomycin, erythromycin and tetracyclines) but not all (chloramphenicol, penicillin) antibiotics.

4. Pyrodoxine (vitamin B-6) supplements reduce the effects of the drug, levodopa, used for treating Parkinson's disease.

5. Vitamin E taken with the blood thinning drug, warfarin, increases the risk of abnormal bleeding. Vitamin E also reduces the body's uptake of the antidepressant, desimpramine.

6. Calcium (carbonate) may interact with Levothyroxine, a drug used to treat thyroid disease and cancer.

In addition, some drugs will affect vitamins and minerals in the body. For example:

1. The cytotoxic antifungal agents, actinomycin and imidazole, may interfere with vitamin D activity.

2. Metaformin is used for treating diabetes and increases the risk of vitamin B-12 deficiency.

CHAPTER 9

EXERCISE

Basic Introduction

DO I REALLY HAVE TO EXERCISE?

WHY BOTHER? Every health article urges us to take regular exercise to become fit thus avoiding **heart problems** and strengthening the bones to prevent age-related diseases such as **osteoporosis** (weakened bones that easily fracture, especially in post-menopausal women). Other benefits from regular exercise are the maintenance of **muscle tone**, the control of **body weight** to lessen the stress on joints, and a reduction in the likelihood of **diabetes** developing. If you suffer from stiffness, weakness and lack of energy, this is not an inevitable consequence of old age (say 50+) but probably due to **inactivity**.

*Advantages of Regular Exercise
Controls body weight
Reduces risk of high blood pressure
Reduces risk of heart problems
Reduces risk of strokes
Reduces risk of diabetes
Strengthens bones
Strengthens resistance to disease
Tones muscles
Increases energy levels

Retains joint flexibility
Increases sexual activity
Delays aging and frailty
Protects against Alzheimer's?
Improves mental outlook
Reduces stress

*See, for example, references 134 and 135

Figure 1, below, shows ABSOLUTELY CLEARLY how a simple exercise such as walking daily can reduce premature death (Graph modified from Hakim and colleagues (see reference 136)

- The graph shows that when retired men walked less than 1 mile per day (< 1 mile) then after 12 years over 40.5% of them had died from all causes. This 40.5% death rate was nearly twice that at 23.8% of another group of retired men who walked more than 2 miles per day (> 2 mile).

- Of these dead men, 13.4% and 5.3% died of cancer, respectively, in the < 1 mile versus the > 2mile groups, while 6.6% and 2.1% died of heart disease/strokes in these same groups.

- In other words, death, cancer and heart disease/stroke rates were 2 to 3 times higher in men who walked less than 1 mile per day compared with those who walked more than 2 miles per day.

Figure 1. Showing how walking regularly can reduce death rates of retired men

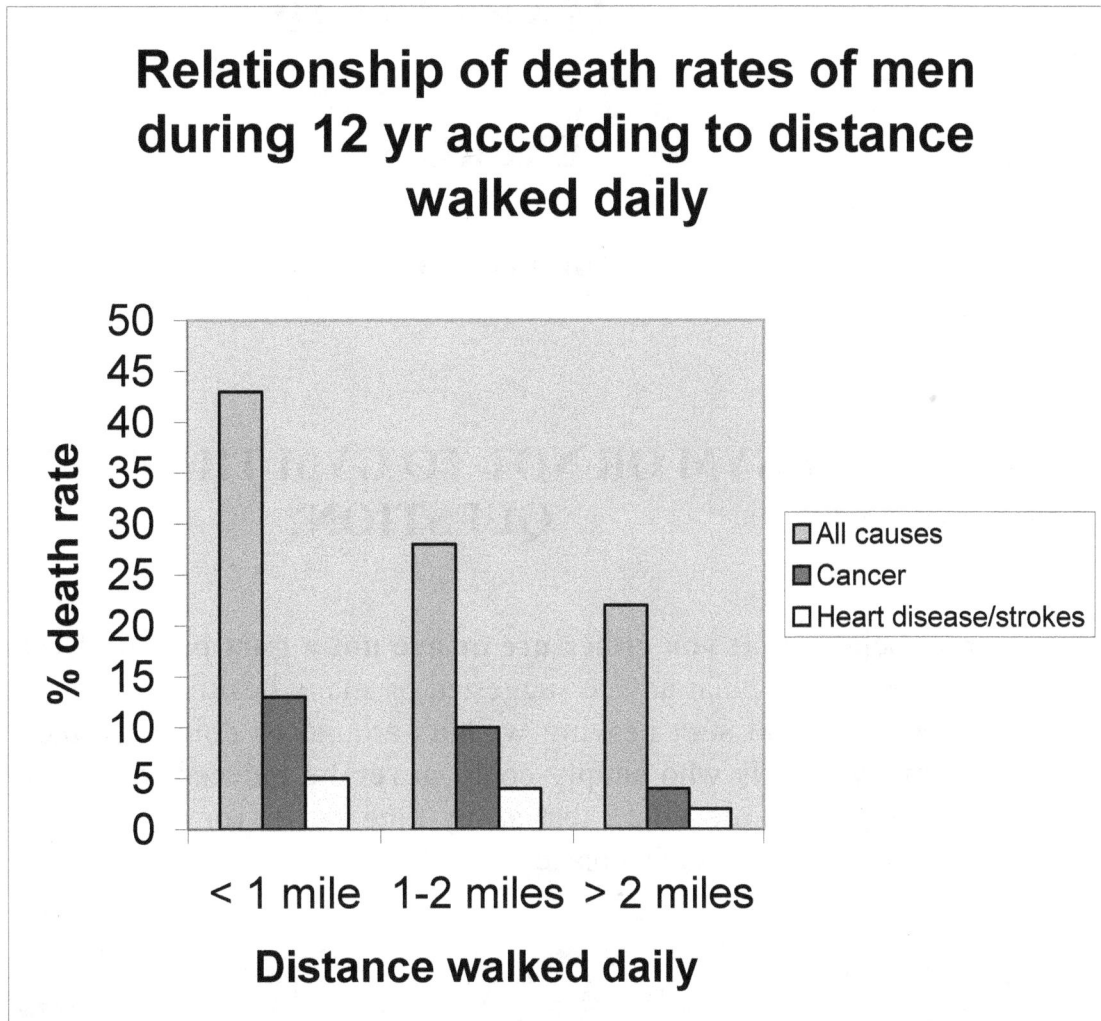

Relationship of death rates of men during 12 yr according to distance walked daily

- You will be amazed how much better you feel once you begin a regular exercise regimen. Regular exercise will help to maintain your mental health and avoid physical problems developing as well as relieving the stress and strain of everyday life.

IT IS ESSENTIAL IF YOU HAVE NOT TAKEN REGULAR EXERCISE FOR A LONG TIME, AND ESPECIALLY IF YOU ARE GROSSLY OVERWEIGHT, THAT YOU CONSULT YOUR DOCTOR BEFORE EMBARKING ON ANY NEW STRENUOUS EXERCISE REGIMEN

CHAPTER 10

EXERCISE

For Gym Lovers

TO GYM OR NOT TO GYM THAT IS THE QUESTION?

- I believe **that you either are or are not a gym person**. Despite this, the most popular advice suggested by many health gurus is **"get ye to a gym"** and start heaving weights around or doing aerobics. I have many friends who simply could **never** be induced to go into a gym and look at me aghast that at my time of life (or any other) I should bother to go to such a place.

- **OK, the gym is not for you.** So miss out this section and go to "Alternative Types of Exercise" (see Chapter 11)

- **For gym people.** Sometimes individuals go to the gym, take one look and never return because they feel **intimidated or self-conscious** in some way. I have visited gyms around the world and can confirm that they are **rarely filled** with perfect physical specimens! Quite the opposite in many cases. So give it a try. **Your first experience** in the gym will very much depend upon the instructor showing you around, as well as the type of gym that you are visiting. Many instructors tend to be young and often very fit and, unfortunately, unaware of the intimidation that can be felt by the novice. They also spend too much time on their stations and not enough keeping an eye on novices using the gym who may be too shy to ask for help.

Figure 1. Avoid gyms full of enormous steroid freaks as you will be intimidated and probably receive scant attention from the instructors

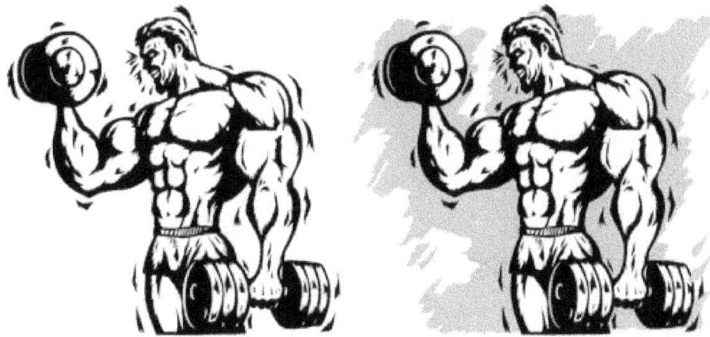

- The **worst type of gym** for a first-timer is where everyone is in their 20-40s, wearing all the latest high–tech gear, and containing a high percentage of posers and/or enormous steroid freaks lifting enormous weights and grunting.

- Try going to **a YMCA or Local Authority Gym** because these tend to contain more of a mix of ages with posers going to the more expensive establishments with larger mirrors all around.

- Try and find someone to train with you as **"Gym Buddies"** are worth their weight in gold and often can correct your technique and provide much-needed motivation. Your gym buddy could be a friend who also wishes to begin training. Believe me, there is nothing like a gym buddy to persuade you to go to the gym on a cold, dark and wet night after a hard days work!

Figure 2. Try and find somebody (your gym buddy) to train with as they will provide motivation and improve your progress

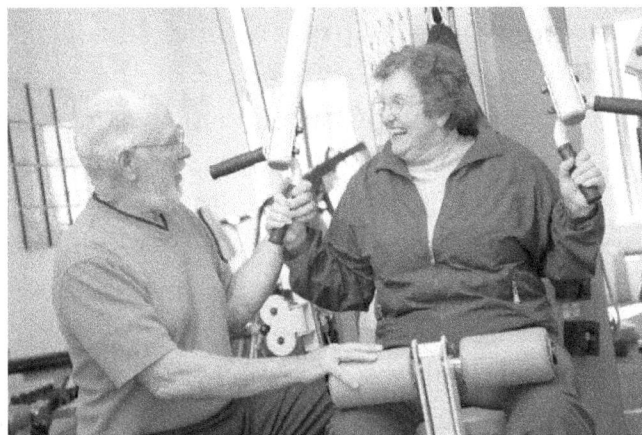

- Ok, you are in the gym at last, so what do you do? One of the instructors should show you how to use all the aerobics equipment (rowing machines, bicycles, treadmills, steppers etc) as well as all the other confusing machines and the free weights (dumbbells and barbells). This is your so-called "**induction**" but don't worry, you will not have to remember everything. Subsequently, he/she **should provide you** with a detailed **written work-out programme** designed uniquely for your requirements. A gym should only allow you to train if you have had an induction in the use of the equipment.

Figure 3. An instructor should show you how to use the equipment (induction) and provide you with a training programme

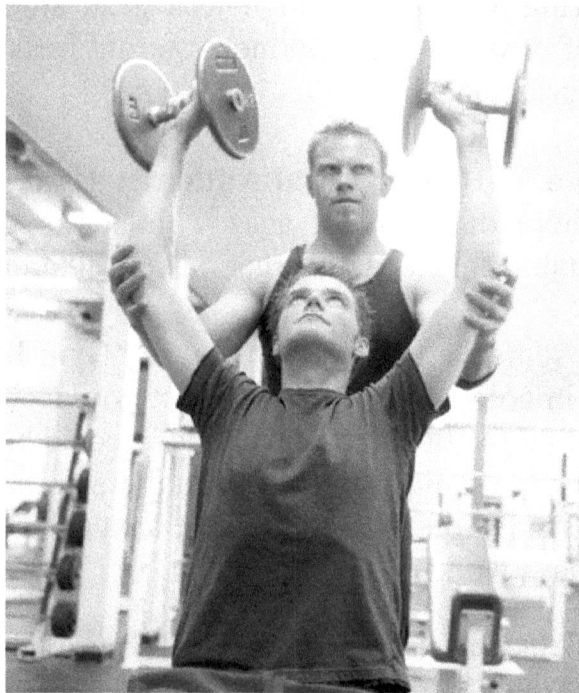

- **Design of your work-out programme.** Ideally, this should contain a mix of aerobic exercise to strengthen the heart, lungs and circulation as well as some weights to strengthen the muscles of the body. The usual advice is to slowly work up to **three 30 minutes aerobic sessions per week** as well as about the same amount of time for weight training. However, these are **just guidelines and should be modified at regular intervals by an instructor**. Personally, I believe that the cycle, rower and the cross trainer (a devilish machine designed to work both the upper body as well as the legs) are better than the treadmill as less impact and wear occurs on the joints.

Aerobic machines can be incredibly **boring** and some gyms run **Cycle Spinning Classes** which involve a semi-circle of static cycles around an instructor on a cycle in the centre who simulates hill climbs and flat racing with you. **Buying a padded seat for these static cycles is advisable**. These spinning classes are good fun and you are usually inspired by an excellent choice of music.

Figure 4. A typical spin class with static cycles

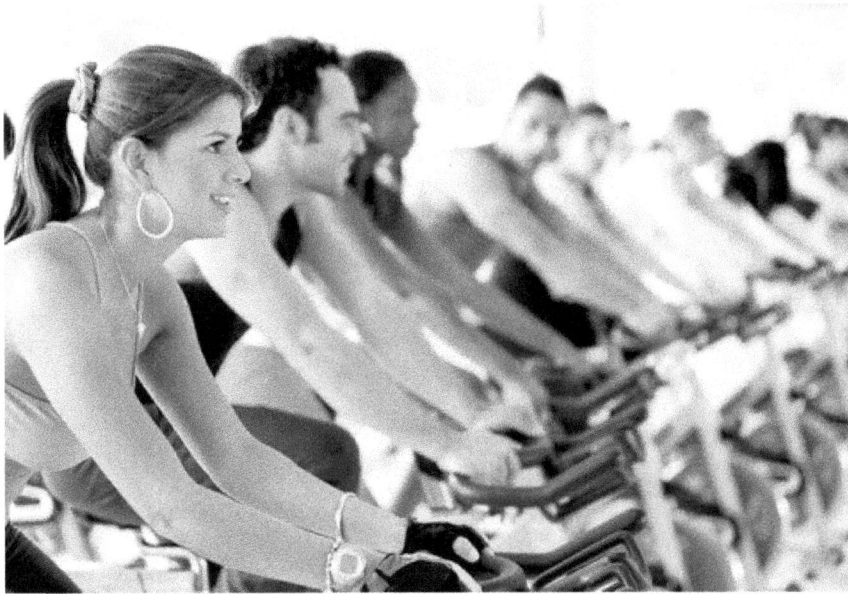

- During the spinning class, you set your own pace (but are actively encouraged by the instructor) and time and calories are rapidly used up. You can burn 800 or more calories in a 50 min session and actually enjoy yourself. A friend of mine once attended a gym in which the cycles had individual screens (like the seats in modern jet planes) on which porno films could be accessed. I guess that he burnt some extra calories in this particular workout! You probably will not have much energy left for weight training after a spinning class so you can do this on another day. However, less strenuous aerobic exercising on the treadmill, bike, rower or cross trainer can be followed by your weight training.

- For starting with weights, if you have not already warmed up with an aerobic session then begin with some gentle aerobic exercise, such as walking or cycling for 5-10 min. Having warmed up, gently, **stretch** the limbs and back, without jerking, as shown in wall charts around the gym and by an instructor. You are now ready to strengthen your body with weights.

Figure 5. Emphasising the necessity of stretching the body prior to strenuous exercise

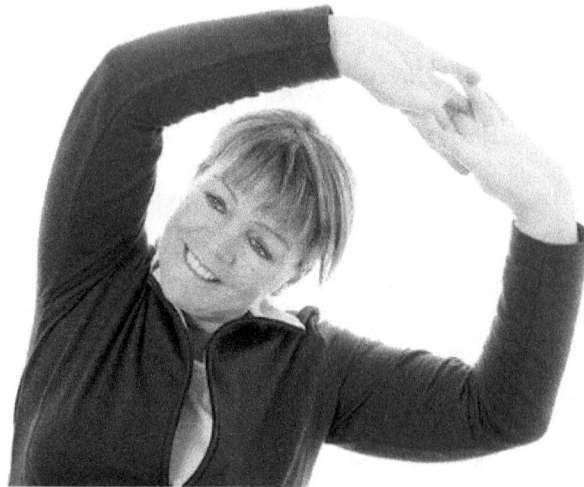

- **Exercising with weights.** First, you have to decide exactly **what you wish to achieve** with the weights. Do you want to generally strengthen the whole body or are there particular parts of your body that you wish to improve?

- **Probably the best strategy** is to train all the main muscle groups in the body each week and then after a few weeks, having mastered your programme and the machines/free weights, fit in some extra repetitions or higher weight to focus on any points of concern such as the abdominals, legs or arms. Again, the instructor should advise you here so do not be frightened to **ask questions**.

- **One possible programme** would be to train Mondays, Wednesdays and Fridays beginning with a 20-30 min aerobic exercise (row, cycle, jog etc) and then followed by a 20-30 min weights session. Finish off by stretching and/or cycling or rowing etc for 5-10 min.

• **Mondays, aerobics then train back and biceps**
• **Wednesdays, aerobics then train chest and abdominal muscles**
• **Fridays, aerobics then train legs, shoulders and triceps**
• **Weekends, walk/cycle or sport** [a]

[a] Try to do some form of exercise at the weekend, even if it is just to stay away from the pub or television for a while. Taking part in some active sport is ideal and can count as an aerobic session. One of the best exercises for ALL AGES is to cycle instead of using the car as this not only burns calories but also saves money and the environment.

- For weights, generally speaking, start with one or two sets of 6+ repetitions and work up to three sets of 10 repetitions with each exercise before increasing the weight.

- For **toning**, the weights should be relatively **light** with higher numbers of repetitions of 15-20. For gaining **muscle bulk,** heavier weights with fewer repetitions of 6-8 should be used. Again, decide which body part you want to improve and ask the instructor to help you.

Things to remember

1. **Always warm up and warm down** for 5-10 min before and after exercise.

2. **Sip water regularly** during your work-out to avoid dehydration and subsequent weakness. Aim to drink about one small bottle of still water, about 500 ml, over a 1-1.5 hour session.

3. Try **not to worry** if you miss one day completely but remember if you feel tired after work then a session in the gym will greatly revitalise you (really).

4. **Muscles adapt** to the same exercise done for week after week so hit the same muscle group with an **alternative exercise** every few weeks.

5. It is very tempting to use heavier and heavier weights after too short a time-the **"MATCHO (macho) EFFECT" (i.e. desire to "match" others lifting big weights in the gym)**. Make sure your **form (your technique) is correct** before you move up the weight otherwise injury can occur.

6. **Do not exercise** if you have a **cold or are ill** as your body is using all its resources to fight the infection and an additional drain on energy sources could be dangerous or even fatal.

7. **Do not exercise shortly after a meal** (within about 1 hour) as all your blood is being used to digest the food rather than being available to the muscles for a sudden workout.

8. **If you feel unwell then stop.** If you still feel unwell some time later consult a doctor.

9. **Do remember to adjust your diet** when you begin training or else you could just stimulate your appetite and put on weight. Again, seek advice from the instructor.

CHAPTER 11

EXERCISE

Alternative Types of Exercise For Gym Haters

These can be undertaken by both **gym-lovers and gym-haters** and have the advantage of reducing or eliminating the need to do aerobic workouts in the gym. The choice of exercises available is enormous and these are summarized in the Table 1 (below) together with the rate at which they burn calories. **Always remember that these figures will vary according to your weight and to the intensity with which you execute the exercise.**

Table 1. ROUGH GUIDE TO CALORIES USED IN VARIOUS TYPES OF EXERCISE BY DIFFERENT WEIGHT PEOPLE.[a]

TYPE OF EXERCISE	CALORIES (kcal) USED PER HOUR WEIGHT (kilos)		
	60	86	102
Gym Activities			
AEROBICS-low impact	359	510	605
BOXING-sparring	575	821	968
CIRCUIT TRAINING	511	730	860
CROSS TRAINING MACHINE	492	700	829
CYCLE MACHINE	447	638	753

ROWING-MACHINE	447	638	753
TREADMILL	492	700	829
SKIPPING-fast	638	912	1075
WEIGHTS-general	184	261	309
WEIGHTS-vigorous	383	547	645
Sports and Hobbies			
BADMINTON [a]	567	805	954
BASKETBALL [a]	511	730	860
CYCLING	511	730	860
DANCING-ballroom	271	386	457
DANCING-modern aerobic	362	514	609
GOLF-carrying bag	325	474	560
HORSERIDING	255	365	430
MARTIAL ARTS	603	857	1017
ROLLERBLADING	447	638	753
ROWING	638	907	1075
RUGBY [a]	606	862	1021
RUNNING-jogging	599	850	1008
SKIING-cross country	487	692	820
SKIING-downhill	391	556	659
SOCCER [a]	575	821	968
SQUASH [a]	816	1092	1248
SWIMMING [a]	383	547	645

TABLE TENNIS [a]	234	340	403
TENNIS-singles [a]	354	504	597
VOLLEYBALL-beach [a]	511	726	860
VOLLEYBALL-gym	241	343	406
WALKING-briskly	263	374	444
WALKING-strolling	184	261	309
YOGA	239	340	403
Home activities			
CLEANING [a]	383	544	645
CLIMBING STAIRS	543	771	914
COOKING-preparation	151	217	257
GARDENING-general [b]	287	431	484
GROCERY SHOPPING	215	306	363
IRONING	136	193	228
PAINTING	303	431	511
SEX [c]	133	189	224
SLEEPING	55	78	92
WATCHING TV	64	91	108
TYPING IN COMPUTER	91	120	203

a. This chart is a general guide since the number of calories you burn will vary according to the intensity of any particular exercise including cleaning. With ball games, this will also depend on your level of expertise and length of rallies or time in play. In addition, the numbers given are those burned by a moderately fit person. Also remember that some of the activities shown, such as sex and climbing stairs, do not usually last for one hour!

b. More active digging and hoeing burn many more calories.

c. Numbers for sex are based on a very optimistic 30 minute session with males burning more calories than females.

THE SNACK WAR

Table 2 explains itself. Many such snacks are not only high in calories but also in harmful fats and gradually reducing these between your main meals would have a significantly beneficial effect on your health by reducing weight and blood pressure. This snack reduction together with an increase or introduction of one or more of the sports in Table 1 **could help avoid many of the diseases associated with aging** such as diabetes and heart attacks. Let us face it, we all eat the odd snack or two and this is no problem if we have a regular exercise routine and our weight is under control.

Table 2. SHOWING THE AMOUNT OF EXERCISE TIME (MINUTES) REQUIRED TO USE UP THE CALORIES PRESENT IN VARIOUS TYPES OF SNACKS [a]

TYPE OF SNACK	CALORIES (kcal) (fat grams)	WALKING	SWIMMING	CYCLING	RUNNING
Cornish Pasty Gingsters (227g)	599 (40.6)	96	66	49	42
Danish pastry	287 (17.4)	46	31	24	20
Doughnut, jam, (75g)	252 (10.9)	40	27	21	18
Flapjack choc chip (85g)	350 (15.5)	56	38	29	25
Galaxy king size	432 (25.2)	69	47	36	30
Geobar (35g)	127 (1.8)	20	14	10	9
Go Ahead Yoghurt break/slice	68 (2.0)	11	7	6	5
Kit Kat (42g)	212 (11.0)	34	23	17	15
Mars Big One (88g)	449 (17.4)	72	49	37	32
Milk Chocolate Dairy whole nut Cadbury (100g)	545 (35.2)	87	60	45	38
Milk Chocolate Digestive Biscuits-2	168 (8.0)	27	18	14	12

Mince-pie (deep-filled)	247	40	27	20	17
Muesli bar (75g)	131 (11.7)	21	14	11	9
Muffin Blueberry Starbucks (100g)	380 (19)	61	41	32	27
Muffin Chocolate Galaxy (86g)	390 (21.8)	62	42	33	28
Pizza Slice Hawaiian	290 (11.0)	47	32	24	20
Popcorn toffee (100g)	408 (7.2)	65	44	34	29
Pot Noodles beef and tomato	378 (14.0)	61	41	31	27
Potato crisps Walkers 50g	263 (14.5)	42	29	22	19
Potato fries (100g)	294 (14.8)	47	32	24	21
Salted Peanuts(50g)	311 (26.5)	50	34	26	22
Sandwich egg and bacon 2 pack	541 (31.3)	87	59	44	38
Sandwich tuna cucumber 2 pack	324 (10.2)	52	36	27	23
SnickersBig One (100g)	501 (28.1)	80	55	41	35
Special K bar (24g)	90 (1.7)	14	10	7	6

a. Based on a someone weighing 86 kilos

Some of the snacks in Table 2 could be substituted, for example by:

1. Fresh or dried fruit (eg. bananas, raisins, sultanas, apricots, prunes, but go easy on the apricots as too many may upset the stomach, also watch out for sulphite preservatives in dried fruit which aggravate allergies). Dates are excellent as they are salt and fat-free but high in fibre, B-vitamins and natural sugar for energy. Each date only contains about 23 calories.

2. A handful of nuts or sunflower or pumpkin seeds (but no more).

3. Unsweetened fruit juice (one glass).

4. Skimmed milk.

5. Small bowl of plain, high fibre, low sugar cereal such as Shredded Wheat, Weetabix or oatmeal with skimmed milk and/or fruit.

6. Plain low fat yoghurt (organic from Sainsbury's is fantastic) with some blueberries, strawberries etc is delicious. Beware of some flavored fruit yoghurts that may contain the artificial sweetener, aspartame, which has recently been reported to induce cancer (see, Table 3 Chapter 5, for details). Frozen yoghurt is a substitute for ice-cream.

7. Boiled eggs occasionally.

8. Rye bread or Ryvita with reduced fat/sugar spread or Marmite.

9. Whole grain, low fat crackers with reduced fat cheese or cottage cheese.

10. Popcorn (98% fat free) or nachos or half a bagel with low fat dip/cheese.

11. Fingers of raw vegetables dipped in low fat dips like hummus etc.

Cravings for sweet snacks may be due to low blood sugar (glucose) resulting from a missed breakfast. Always eat breakfast and include food, such as porridge, cereal or wholemeal toast that release glucose slowly into the blood.

NOW LET'S BEGIN TO EXERCISE

TRUE STORIES SHOWING HOW **NOT** TO BEGIN

Case 1

Is a middle-aged man of 42 who had never been interested in the gym or sport but had begun to put on weight around his waist. He decided to start running to control his weight gain. He failed to ask advice regarding a training schedule but just put on his daps and took off at **high speed** down the hill outside his home. After about one mile, he turned around and started running uphill back to his house. He eventually arrived home exhausted and gasping for breath. The next day massive stiffness set in and he could hardly walk. This was such a traumatic experience that he **never ran** or tried any active exercise again up to now, 15 years later.

Case 2

Involved a 34 year old man who decided to play squash after a **two year lay-off**. The game was very competitive and shortly after finishing he complained of pins and needles in his arms and was unable to breathe properly. He ended up in hospital only to be told by the doctor that another man had died a few days previously on the same squash court! Fortunately, he recovered but **never again participated** in any active sport.

The moral of these stories is to **BEGIN SLOWLY** and select activities that you enjoy and that will retain your enthusiasm. The idea is to increase your daily physical activity not to break a world record. What exactly was the purpose of the runner in Case 1 above? He failed to achieve anything although he could possibly have set a new world speed record for having a heart attack!

THE SENSIBLE WAY

Select some activity that you have or previously had **an interest** in. This could include:

1. Joining a football, rugby, running, tennis, bowls or cycling club – anything to keep you away from the television couch.

2. Qualifying as a football or rugby referee or coach.

3. Learning or improving your swimming or gaining a diving qualification which will open a whole new world to you under the sea.

4. **OR just increasing an activity that you are already involved in** such as walking the dog more often or for a longer time at a faster pace. A study showed that a 20 minute walk with the dog 5 times per week can result in weight loss of 14 lbs in one year. Walking is easy as you need no special training or equipment, although a good pair of shoes/trainers is essential, and you are unlikely to suffer injury. Since many people are goal orientated then why not buy a pedometer to motivate you to achieve the recommended 10,000 paces per day?

Whatever activity you chose, try and involve a friend as, like the "gym buddy" (in Chapter 10), you can motivate each other on a cold dark night to leave the house and exercise. After all, friends are excellent for motivating us to go and drink in the pub.

Some people who hate both exercise and the gym have found that buying a pull-up bar over the door, some dumbbells and an aerobic workout machine, such as a treadmill or a cycle/rowing machine, for their homes is the answer. If you are a novice to using this equipment then ask a friend for help or enroll for a free induction week at a nearby gym. A good animated website for dumbbell workouts at home is **www.sport-fitness-advisor.com/dumbbellexercises.html**. The advantages and disadvantages of the aerobic machines are:

- Their use is independent of the weather

- You can watch the television

- You can record the time, distance, calories burned and pulse rate each day and monitor your progress

- **However,** I have noticed that after a while, these machines tend to become "invisible" and disappear into the rest of the furniture or end up rusting on the patio!

- There are also many other distractions at home such as children, pets, housework etc.

It is up to you to decide whether you wish to confine your exercise to the home or bite the bullet and expose your body to the outside world

Probably, an important consideration is **your location**. Thus, if you live in a dangerous inner city and cannot stand the gym then you have little choice but to remain at home unless you are prepared to drive out of town. On the other hand if, like me, you are lucky enough to live by the sea then you can feel safe in the company of other joggers running along the promenade.

The other advantage of exercising outside is that you will soon see other people jogging with **worse** weight/fitness problems than yourself.

How many times per week?

As mentioned above (see Chapter 10 on the GYM), exercising three times per week for at least 30 minutes is a realistic goal just for the aerobic part of your programme. **DO REMEMBER,** however, that although cycling, running, and football will tone your legs, stomach, heart and lungs, they will do little to maintain your **upper body musculature** and retain a balanced physique. That is why many athletes and sports people include some sort of weight training that not only balances their physiques but also strengthens the whole body and improves their overall performance.

I have often seen it recommended to exercise five times per week (by Medical Officers, no less) to ward off ill-health and obesity. Yes, exercising every day would be ideal but we have to be realistic and set achievable goals. Starting any new programme of exercise, even once or twice per week, is a major effort for some people so let us aim for three sessions per week and take it from there. Three exercise sessions combined with some of the dietary recommendations made above (see Chapter 1) will rapidly produce results and be self-fulfilling. It will not only produce pleasing and obvious physical changes but also increased mental alertness and feelings of well-being. These in turn will reinforce the benefits of a new life style and help avoid slipping back to previous self-destructive ways. In addition, trying to exercise five or more times per week will often involve major changes to daily routines, in already busy lives, that are impossible to maintain.

Also, the **amount of exercise required** will depend upon your age, weight, calorie intake and your present level of activity each day. **It is possible to increase** your exercise level each day simply by using the stairs instead of the lift, by walking/cycling into work or by cleaning the house more regularly.

Do remember that exercise will stimulate your appetite

Case 3

I have a number of friends with weight problems who regularly exercise but never seem to shed their "pot bellies". Only by following their eating and drinking habits did I find out why. One friend was very fond of Indian meals and after exercising went to the local Indian restaurant which served "all you can eat" dinners. I joined him on several occasions and although I burnt twice as many calories as him in the gym, he ate **twice as much food as I did!** Another friend regularly ran 3-4 times per week for at least 30 minutes per day. He always seemed to be on the treadmill covered in sweat. He weight trained too but always looked out-of-condition in the changing room. His problem was simply that the exercise seemed to be stimulating his thirst for beer which he drank in large amounts many an evening. One pint of lager with about 200 calories would have taken him at least 15 minutes to jog away and I am sure that he had more than just 2-3 pints in a night.

CHOICE OF DIFFERENT EXERCISES AND SPORTS

The choice of different exercises available seems almost endless but some of the most common ones are listed in Table 1 (above) and the basic characteristics of the most common exercises are given in Table 3 (below). These exercises seem to fall into various categories, namely:

1. Team sports such as rugby, soccer, volleyball, hockey, cricket and basketball

2. Individual or doubles sports such as badminton, squash, tennis, table tennis, cycling, walking, running, skiing, horse riding, swimming, surfing, rollerblading, martial arts, yoga and golf

3. Hobbies/housework such as gardening, cooking, cleaning, decorating and shopping

4. Sex

5. Exercise for lazy or hectic people

1. Team Sports (Table 3)

Most of these are ideal for maintaining fitness of people in their teens, 20s and 30s and up to the beginning of middle age. **I leave individuals to decide when middle age begins!** In contact team sports, especially such as rugby, soccer and basketball, the time to look around for alternative ways to stay fit is usually indicated by recurrent injuries that take ages to heal. Older rugby players sometimes recognize the march of time and play a modified game called "touch rugby" with none of the usual vigorous body tackling allowed.

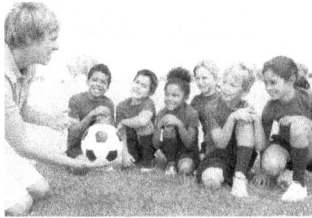

Rugby, soccer and basketball

These require high levels of all-round fitness involving sprinting and high levels of endurance. Different degrees of fitness are required according to the position played. Rugby, soccer and basketball players all benefit from strength training involving weights. With rugby, the emphasis is on all round power, strength and flexibility involving bench pressing and squats. Soccer and basketball players also train with weights to strengthen their legs and maximize vertical jumping ability. Care must be taken not to lose leg strength during endurance training.

2. Common Individual or Doubles Sports (Table 3)

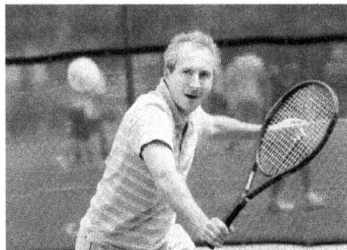

Racket sports

Badminton, squash, tennis and table tennis are sports that can be taken up as children and continued throughout life, even into the 70s and beyond. Care must be taken to avoid injuries to the joints caused by incorrect footwear or racket grip as well as injuries to the eyes or head from squash balls or rackets. Warm-up and warm-down routines are also essential to avoid muscle and joint problems. **Squash, in particular, can be extremely**

strenuous and should not be played by unfit, overweight, middle–aged people, new to the sport, without clearance from the doctor.

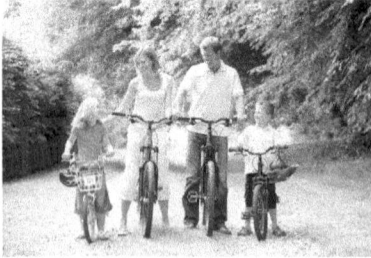

Cycling

This is the most wonderful and exhilarating sport/past-time undertaken by young and old alike. It has the advantage over walking and running in that greater distances are covered more rapidly and the frequent scenery changes maintain interest. Cycling is also a practical replacement for the car/local transport for travelling to work. An even more important advantage of cycling is that it is a low-impact activity that **does little damage to the joints**. Cycling is weight bearing when standing on the pedals for riding up hills (refer to Table 3). Disadvantages are the increased risk of accidents and pollution on busy roads. In addition, there are reports that too frequent cycling for long distances can cause fertility and impotence problems. Reduced sperm counts may result from overheating of the testicles in tight shorts and temporary impotence may be caused by constant pressure from the saddle decreasing the blood flow to the penis. Reduction in excessive bike riding has been advised, in some cases, during attempts to start a family. Padded, gel-containing seat covers offer protection too. Make sure that you cycle about 5 times the distance that you would walk or run. Ensure that you maintain a rhythm sufficient to raise your pulse but can still answer questions from companions-the so-called **"talk-test"**. Finally, do not cycle for a few days prior to the "prostate specific antigen" (PSA) test, which should be undergone by all 50+ year old males every year, as cycling can elevate PSA levels.

Walking

We all walk every day but simply by increasing your walking time each day you can increase your fitness level. Walking is also low impact and weight bearing to strengthen the bones (Table 3). Walk to the shops or to work and take the children to school on foot rather than by car. Walking the dog or with a friend are great ways of increasing your daily exercise. Many of my friends walk to work or at lunchtime and have noticed the difference in their fitness levels after just a few weeks, even though they do no other form of exercise. Recently, it has been recommended that we aim for 10,000 steps each day. Frankly, this sounds ridiculous for busy people to achieve but apparently most people already take 3-5,500 steps per day. I believe that the weather in the UK does not encourage walking but buying a pedometer to record the daily steps can motivate some people. **The 10,000 steps correspond to the minimum level required per day to achieve the benefits of regular exercise.** Some people will prefer to walk indoors on a treadmill away from the rain and cold and can easily record their progress while watching the TV. Gradually increase the time and pace at which you walk and remember the **"talk-test"** to monitor your work intensity. Make sure that you have comfortable shoes appropriate for the terrain.

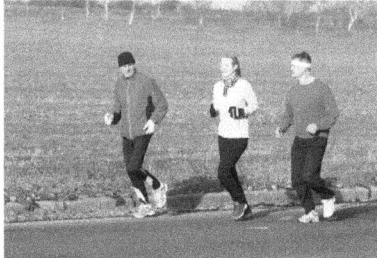

Running and jogging

Running is probably **the most effective way of achieving cardiovascular fitness** and is a major component of many sports. In addition, running at a slower speed (jogging) can be utilized by itself to achieve maximal fitness. Like walking, you can easily adjust your programme to suit your needs and can jog when and where you please. Some people begin by jogging short distances after years of inactivity and end up running marathons! The great advantage of jogging is that it burns calories more rapidly than walking and takes less time. The disadvantage of jogging is that it is **high impact (Table 3) and without good running shoes can damage the joints, especially if you are overweight**. When starting, after years of inactivity, consult your doctor before you begin. If you are unfit and overweight then begin by walking for a short time and then gradually increase your speed until you can run slowly and maintain a conversation **(talk test again)**. Do not worry if progress is slow, but aim to build up the time rather than the distance run, until you can run 20-30 minutes for three times per week. **Do remember to jog in a safe area frequented by other people and try and vary your routine.** Ideally, use a sports centre and run with other people at about the same level of fitness as yourself. Always warm up slowly before running and stretch afterwards.

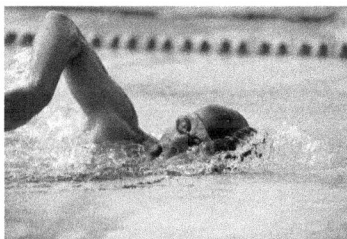

Swimming

Is a marvellous form of general exercise and works out almost **every major muscle group** in the body and increases stamina, strength and flexibility. Swimming also has **low impact** as the water supports the body and there is little stress on any of the joints. Since swimming is not a weight-bearing exercise (Table 3), it does little to strengthen the bones and protect against osteoporosis. It is therefore a good idea to **combine swimming with some weight-bearing exercise** such as walking, running or gym work (Table 3). Swimming is also a good fat-burning exercise and is ideal for people with arthritis, back problems and degenerative diseases as well as pregnant women. The water supports the body, reduces the body weight and allows people to exercise who would normally not be able to because of problems with their joints and back. Swimming is also **excellent for the heart and lungs** since increasing your speed will result in a superb aerobic workout that can easily be undertaken 3 or more times per week. Varying the stroke from backstroke to crawl to breaststroke will also ensure that the majority of muscles in the body are exercised. The value of exercising in water is reflected by the use of swimming pools by many hospital physiotherapists for the treatment of patients with arthritic and other conditions. Regarding the use of swimming for weight loss, there is evidence that swimming is less effective than running or cycling for reducing weight. This may be related to swimming enhancing appetite more than most aerobic activities due to the cooling affect of the water on the body. Again, it is obvious that **all exercise will stimulate the appetite and this urge to eat more has to be controlled.**

Final Comment on Sports

The above sports have the greatest appeal for people wishing to get fit at all ages. This is due to the lack of specialist training required, in most cases, to participate and the wide availability of places to undertake them. **Not all of these activities are suitable for everyone** as evidenced, for example, by my own inability to master swimming beyond a couple of lengths of frantic activity to stay afloat! The important thing is to **find an activity that you enjoy and which you are happy to do three or more times per week** in order to remain fit. Many other sports, such as rowing and skiing, have not been detailed as they require specialist training, equipment or facilities.

3/4. Hobbies/Housework and Sex (Table 3)

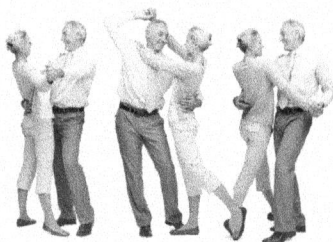

Dancing

Probably one of the **best hobbies** for obtaining and maintaining fitness for the very young and into old age is dancing. Dancing includes ballroom, ballet, square, disco, jazz, jiving, pole and Latin American as well as belly dancing and aerobic workouts, all of which **greatly benefit the heart and lungs and improve flexibility, co-ordination, strength and stamina (Table 3)**. Dancing is also very sociable and helps to find friends and partners. Many events for single people often involve regular meetings for dancing and talking. It was a great relief for me and many of my friends when **disco dancing finally arrived**, as it allowed us to participate without the need to learn prescribed steps or have any degree of co-ordination. Thus, without any training, you can meet members of the opposite sex, have aerobic conditioning and tone the body. The disadvantages include the fact that **many people drink and smoke (not in UK now)** at dance venues. In discos, women also usually benefit more than men who tend to huddle together in groups watching the women!

Exercise/dance or aerobic videos

These videos are also helpful for people (usually women) who **hate the gym or exercising outdoors and prefer to exercise at home**. You can find videos for any type of work-out from yoga to aerobics and dance. Beware videos made by show-biz, usually female, celebrities who have dropped a few dress sizes and are trying to make a fast buck. One of the most ridiculous videos was made by a soap star who lost weight and made a video, then put the weight back on, only to shed it again and make another video! Remember, many videos available are made by fit, good-looking, young women who, lets face it, should be fit at their age. Look under **www.videofitness.com** for a review of videos but **beware those using rapid, high impact, step aerobics**, as without careful instruction on speed, technique and step height, you can easily injure knees and other joints.

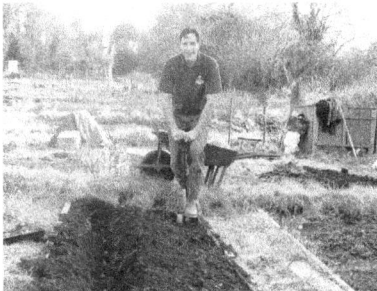

Gardening

Gardening can be a wonderful way of keeping fit but only if activities are included to elevate the pulse and breathing rates (Table 3). It is no use just sowing a few seeds or pruning the roses and expecting to stay fit. In order to stimulate the heart rate, try mowing the lawn using a manual lawn mower, aerating the lawn manually with a fork or digging the vegetable patch. Sawing and chopping are also excellent exercises that can be incorporated. Apart from the fact that it is outside, the great advantage of gardening is the huge satisfaction and health benefits of harvesting your own vegetables and fruit, as well as the shear pleasure of viewing that well-trimmed lawn and colourful flower beds.

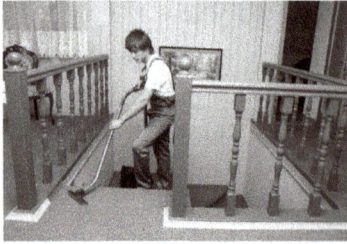

Housework

Personally, I can think of nothing worse than having to rely on housework to assist in remaining fit. It is possible, however, for parents with jobs, and little spare time, to incorporate housework into their fitness programme. Such activities as vacuuming, scrubbing, washing and climbing the stairs will raise the pulse and can be executed with some background music to help maintain a rhythm and pass the time. Remember to elevate the heart rate for at least 20 minutes for optimal effects.

Sex

There is no disputing that exercise is good for the sex life but sex is unlikely to make a major impact on your fitness programme. Regular exercising increases strength, stamina and flexibility all of which will benefit your sex life. In addition, exercise stimulates the release of testosterone and enhances the sex drive. Men who exercise and control their weight also have more active sex lives and less erectile problems.

Table 3. BASIC CHARACTERISTICS OF DIFFERENT EXERCISES

Exercise	Ideal ages	Cardio vascular training	Weight-bearing	Impact	Joint damage	Other injuries	Advantages/ disadvantages
Teams, rugby, soccer etc	Teens-30s	Very good	Yes, variable	Yes	Common	Very common	Injuries accumulate
Racket sports	Any	Very good	Yes, legs	Yes	Very common	Sometimes	Joint wear and tear
Cycling	Any	Very good	Yes, if standing	Low	Low	May reduce fertility	Great distances, pollution/ accident risks
Walking	Any	Fair	Yes, legs	Low	Low	Uncommon	Slow but favored by elderly
Running/ jogging	Teens to 40/50s	Very good	Yes, legs	High	Common	Uncommon	Safety problem in cities

Swimming	Any	Very good	No	None	None	Uncommon	May also need weight bearing exercise
Dancing	Any	Low-Variable	Yes, legs	Yes	Variable	Uncommon	Sociable but smoking and drinking
Gardening	20s +	Low-Variable	Yes, variable	Yes	Variable	Cuts	Outside, relaxing, produces vegetables/ flowers
Housework	20s +	Low-Variable	Yes, variable	Low	Variable	Sometimes	Boring, can be dangerous

OR IS THE FOLLOWING YOU?

5. Exercise for Lazy, Stressed or Hectic People

Despite the vast media exposure of the benefits of a weekly exercise programme, **many people still do very little each day**.

Figure 1. Man overcome by laziness and unaware of long-term harm of his inactive lifestyle

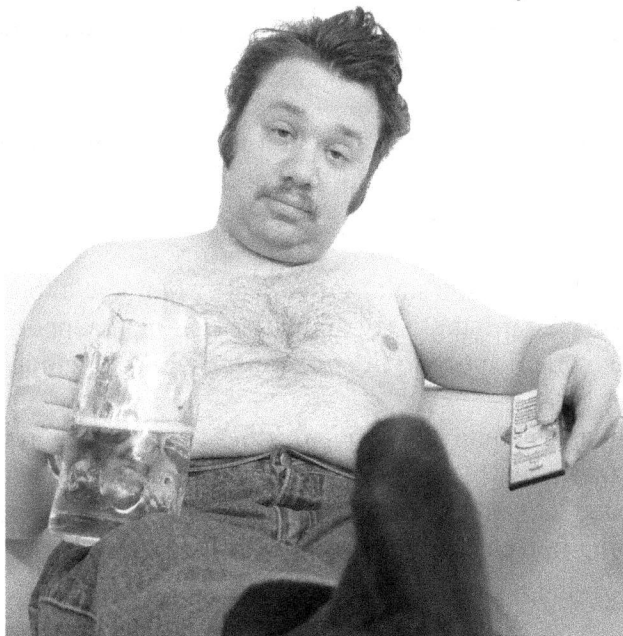

This lack of exercise may be due to:

- **laziness** and lack of concern about their health

- **depression** or excessive stress associated with family/financial problems

- **extremely hectic** lifestyles

The Chartered Association of Physiotherapy have produced an excellent booklet entitled **"The Lazy Exercise Guide"** that may help these groups of people (see reference 137). This booklet explains how daily activities can be modified to provide some sort of workout. **This, however, should be seen only as a stop-gap until time allows for a more organized exercise programme.** In addition, the advice below is also valuable for people who regularly work out. The guide is divided into sections some of which are modified here:

1. **Beginning the day** use the towel to dry your back diagonally from hip to shoulder to provide both a stretch and muscular toning. Stretch legs, arms and neck while dressing.

2. **Journeying** to work in the car and sitting with a straight back and exercising the pelvic floor muscles (abdominal workout and may reduce impotence in men too (see reference 138). On the bus or train, adjust the posture with shoulders back, tummy in and stand as tall as possible. Also, get off one stop earlier and walk to and from work, using the stairs instead of the lift whenever possible in work.

3. **In work** leave your desk every 20 minutes and walk around and stretch the back and legs.

4. **Lunching,** some people use this time for fresh air and a walk, maybe bringing in sandwiches (healthy home made!) and walking to the park. Again concentrate on your posture and walk tall pulling in the tummy.

5. **At home,** walk around or up and down the stairs at every TV commercial break or get up from the computer every 20 minutes. Try and sit upright and support your back at all times. You can also practice pelvic floor exercises while watching TV.

6. **Housework,** activities such as vacuum cleaning, dusting and ironing provide excellent opportunities for additional exercise. Move the furniture around but make sure that you bend your legs when lifting. Play some music and clean in time to this with long sweeping movements and again with the tummy drawn in.

7. **Social events,** again much of the above apply when travelling by car or public transport. It is an excellent idea to try and walk home after a meal rather than catching a taxi. This will help digestion and sleeping.

All the above sounds slightly ridiculous but is just trying to help you to begin some exercise before it is too late. In reality, if you are that lazy or depressed nothing will motivate you and you will not be reading this book.

EXERCISING AT DIFFERENT AGES

It cannot be stated too strongly just how **vitally important it is to undertake some form of exercise throughout life** in order to maintain both physical and mental health. Recent research has shown that as well as the general population, children from **the age of 2 and even people in their 70s, 80s or even 90s benefit** as well as Alzheimer's patients. As mentioned previously, the type of exercise undertaken will vary according to your age.

- **Children**

Numbers of obese children has risen steadily over the last 20-25 years. A 2005 report from the Governments Information Statistics Division revealed that Scottish children were the fattest in the world with 34% overweight and nearly 20% obese. The later, 2007-2009, rates are very similar for children in the whole UK with 32.6% overweight and 18.3% obese at 10-11 yrs old, and seem to have peaked in the last few years (see reference 139). Unfortunately, overweight and sedentary children tend to develop into overweight adults. These in turn will have higher incidences of bowel cancer, high blood pressure, heart attacks, strokes and type 2 diabetes. The problem of being overweight/obesity needs to be **tackled in children less than 11 years of age before a pattern of poor diet and lack of exercise is developed**. Over 40% of children more than 6 years old may not be exercising for the 30-60 min per day recommended. This is because of the vast amount of time spent in front of the TV and computer, and due to the fact that they do not walk to school or participate regularly in sport.

Increase your children's exercise by:

1. Walking with them to the shops.

2. Buying them a bicycle or skates.

3. Taking them regularly to the park for soccer, basketball, cricket etc.

4. Teaching them to swim in the local sports centre.

5. Buying them a dog but only if they agree to walk it every day.

6. Finding out about the amount of physical activity and sport offered at school and becoming involved as a volunteer coach, referee, sponsor etc.

7. Reducing the amount of time they use the computer or spend watching the television each day.

8. Acting as a role model and regularly exercising yourself.

You may soon find that your children's school work, mental health, weight and sleep patterns improve. You too will get more exercise on the touchline or out with the dog.

- **Teens and twenties**

These are the optimal ages for the type of exercise demanding explosive muscular movements and contact sports. The body is more resilient and flexible and less likely to suffer injury. When injury does occur, the healing process is much more rapid than at later ages. Thus, this is the **best time for soccer, rugby, boxing, skiing, gymnastics, martial arts, basketball and many athletics events**, and is the reason that professionals in most of these sports peak by the time they are 30. This does not mean that the average person should not pursue these sports after 30 but, if they do, then they will be more prone to injury.

Many men in their twenties, who do not participate in the above-   mentioned sports, tend to **neglect their cardiovascular workouts** and head for the gym to heave heavy weights around. Reasons for this are fuelled by pressure from society to have the perfect physique both for self fulfillment and for the attraction of the opposite sex. This is apparent from the role models seen in pop videos in which the men with bulging muscles are often surrounded by scantily dressed women. This would be fine if it was not for the great temptation to take shortcuts offered by steroids that are now widely used in some gyms.

This age-group should therefore ensure that they incorporate sufficient aerobic exercise into their gym routines in the form of team sports and/or running, cycling outdoors or aerobic machine work in the gym.

In this age group, particularly, both men and women need to develop an exercise regimen as part of their normal daily routine. Exercise will then be seen as a normal component of their lifestyle and incorporated into later years with minimal effort. This is vitally important since during the late twenties, if not before (see below, "Sarcopenia", for more details), muscles that are not regularly exercised will begin to shrink and fat deposits will begin to build up.

Not as many women as men participate in team sports, and gyms often contain many more men than women. Unfortunately, some women have also adopted men's drinking habits without offsetting these bad habits with regular exercise regimes. The consequences are obvious with increasing numbers of young women overweight.

- **Thirties to forties**

This is the time during which contact sports become replaced with exercises designed to retain physical strength and optimal cardiovascular functioning.

> **There are two particular problems that can become apparent after 35-40 years of age. These are:**

1. Loss of muscle mass – called **"sarcopenia"** – (see Figure 2, below) which results in increasing weakness and frailty (see reference 140). It has been estimated that after 45 years old, muscle mass declines about 0.5-1% per year up to 60. Muscle loss then accelerates throughout the 60s, 70s and 80s, and, eventually, results in frailty and the inability to carry out simple daily tasks.

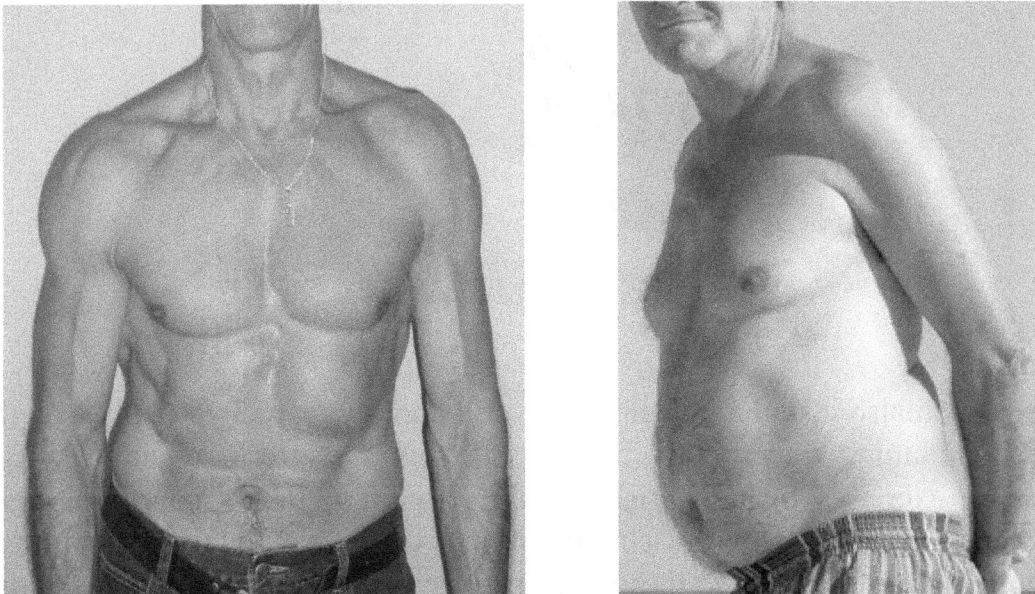

Figure 2. Showing the bodies of two middle aged men. In the right hand photo, it is obvious that some loss of muscle mass has occurred in the upper arms and shoulders and that muscle has been replaced by fat elsewhere. The man in the left photo has used weights to prevent the effects of sarcopenia

2. Thinning and weakening of the bones – called **"osteoporosis"** – which results in increased likelihood of fractures from minor falls. With osteoporosis, calcium is lost from the bones and if the vertebrae of the spine are affected, and become compressed, then people can shrink remarkably in height.

Both sarcopenia and osteoporosis can, however, be prevented, at least partially, in the 30-40s with weight-bearing exercises. *The best weight-bearing exercises are those using dumbbells, barbells or resistance machines in the gym.* These can easily be substituted for by doing press-ups or other exercises using the body weight or by buying a set of dumbbells for use in the home. The weights should be used 2 or 3 times per week and at each time 9-10 sets of exercises should be done containing 6 to 10 repetitions in each set.

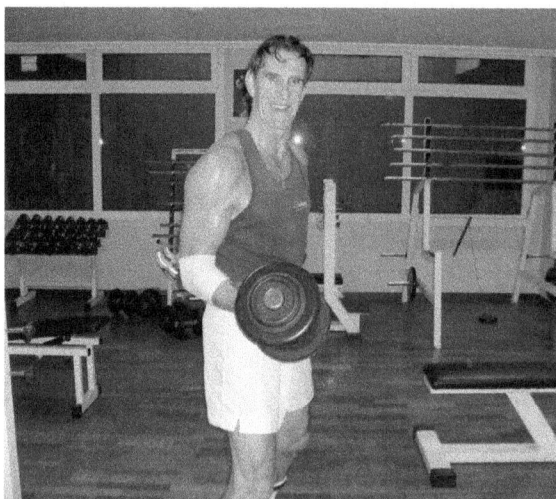

Many men also install a pull-up bar over a doorway which is really excellent for maintaining upper body strength in this age group. Gentler weight-bearing exercises include brisk walking, running, racket sports, skipping, dancing, backpacking, cross-country skiing, volley ball, as well cleaning and digging in the garden. Do these 2-3 times per week for 20-30 min each time. Many of these are excellent as they also provide the required amount of cardiovascular exercise needed each week. The value of swimming as a non-weight bearing, cardiovascular exercise for all ages cannot be over-emphasized but is ineffective at preventing sarcopenia and osteoporosis.

- **Fifties, sixties and beyond**

Having incorporated exercise into your normal weekly regimen, **there is no reason why this should not be continued into the 50s, 60s and beyond**. There are now more and more people participating in tennis and squash tournaments beyond 65 years old as well as older and older marathon runners reported in the press.

Tennis and walking seem particularly suited for continuation beyond the 60s as they do not require violent bursts of speed and the risk of falls is therefore limited. The normal routines of the younger years can therefore be continued unless overweight, heart disease, high blood pressure, diabetes or arthritis have taken an excessive toll. Hopefully, none of these will apply to readers of this book who have followed the advice offered.

With people living longer, there is more time for them to incorporate regular cardiovascular and weight-bearing exercise into their lives. **Swimming is excellent** for the heart and lungs, and for maintaining flexibility and co-ordination in the older athlete. The value of swimming for the elderly has recently been recognized by Health Challenge Wales and across the UK by the introduction of free swimming for the over 60s. As detailed in the "30s to 40s" section (above), *it is vital to undertake resistance training (weight training), as well as exercises for the heart and lungs*, to avoid **sarcopenia or muscle wasting**. Without resistance training, **sarcopenia** will accelerate in the 60s, 70s and 80s resulting in the **"Frailty Syndrome"** with an increasing inability to carry out daily jobs around the house. An elderly person with advanced sarcopenia may even find it impossible to rise from a chair. This physical weakness will lead to disability and dependency on others as routine tasks are neglected. **"The downward spiral of aging" therefore accelerates and the care home will be the only solution as the person can no longer maintain an independent life.**

The important message is that even very unfit elderly people can benefit from an exercise programme, providing there are no major health problems. Unbelievable increases in strength by lifting weights have even been reported for people as old as 90.

IT IS VITAL, FOR MAINTAINING INDEPENDENCE IN OLDER PEOPLE, TO PRESERVE MUSCULAR STRENGTH, COORDINATION AND FLEXIBILITY IN ORDER TO CARRY OUT SIMPLE DAILY TASKS AROUND THE HOME, SUCH AS CLIMBING THE STAIRS, CLEANING AND PREPARING FOOD

NB. IT IS NEVER TOO LATE TO BEGIN SOME STRENGTHENING EXERCISES – EVEN IN YOUR EIGHTIES

For example, my 86 year old neighbour began exercising, while sitting in her armchair, some very light strengthening exercises for her arms using very small dumbells or weights attached to her wrists with Velcro. After 3 months, she was delighted to be able to lift up her grandchildren to kiss them, for the very first time, as well as to regain her ability to turn her light switches on and off.

Figure 3. Showing the author's elderly neighbour using dumbbells to strengthen arms and shoulders

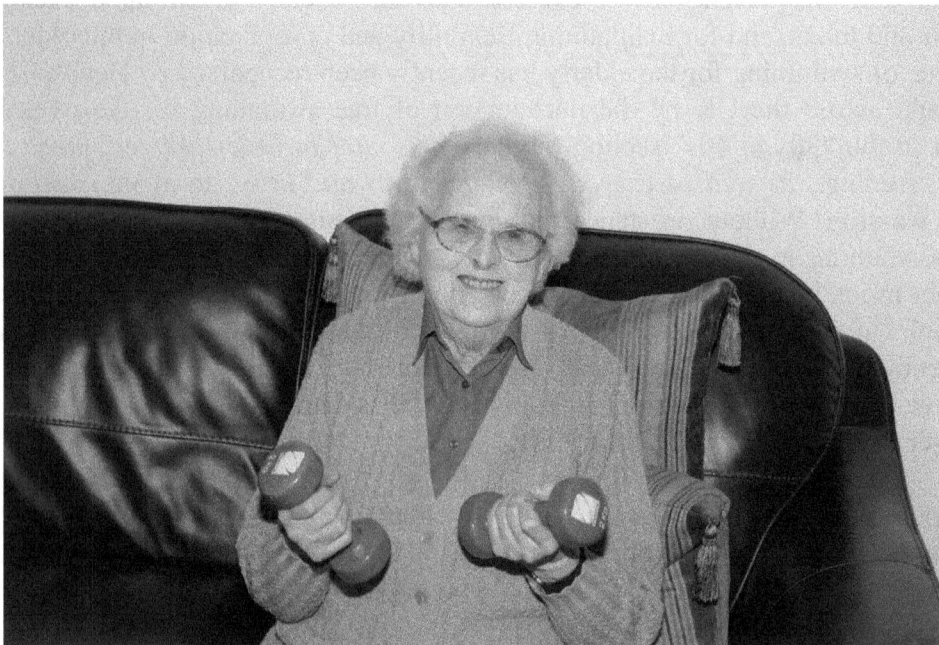

Sarcopenia can, thus, be treated and prevented to a large extent without the use of drugs. These same resistance exercises will also help to protect against osteoporosis (bone thinning).

There is no need to join a gym as light weights are inexpensive to buy and household objects, such as plastic bottles filled with sand or water, are just as effective. A basic home weight resistance programme and exercises for the elderly can be found in reference 141. Such simple programmes not only strengthen the arms, but also the legs in order to prevent falls.

Results can be very impressive with significant increases in both muscle mass and strength recorded even for residents of care homes.

For the latest health advice go to:

http://endtheconfusion.wordpress.com

APPENDIX

Reference sources for conclusions made in each chapter

Chapter 1

1. Giovannucci and colleagues. A prospective study of tomato products, lycopene, and prostate cancer risk. Journal National Cancer Institute, Vol. 94, pages 391–398, 2002.
2. Kavanaugh and colleagues, Journal of the National Cancer Institute, Vol. 99, pages 1074-1085, 2007.
3. Sinha and colleagues, Archives of Internal Medicine, Vol. 169, pages 562-571, 2009.
4. Bochukova, and colleagues. Large, rare chromosomal deletions associated with severe early-onset obesity. Nature 6th December, 2009 (http://dx.doi.org/10.1038/nature08689).
5. www.salt.gov.uk/publications.html for a free download of "The Little Book of Salt".
6. Draft Energy Requirements report 'scientific consultation', SACN, November 2009.

Chapter 2

7. www.eatwell.gov.uk/foodlabels/trafficlights
8. www.weightlossresources.co.uk/calories-in-food
9. www.calorieking.com/foods
10. www.tiscali.co.uk/lifestyle/healthfitness/calorie/data
11. Lee and Griffin, Nutrition Bulletin, Vol.31, pages 21-27, 2006.
12. "Fit Not Fat at 40+" (Prevention Health Books, 2004, published by Rodale Inc. (ISBN1-4050-4179-X).

Chapter 3

13. Perspectives in Public Health, Vol. 129, pages 56-57, 2009 (see: http://rsh.sagepub.com)
14. www.atkinsexposed.org for detailed refs on the Atkins Diet.
15. Gardner and colleagues, J. American Medical Association, Vol. 297, pages 969-977, 2007.
16a. Govindji, A. and N. Puddefoot, "The 10-Day Gi Diet", published by Vermillion, UK, 2006.

Chapter 4

16b. www.foodsafetymagazine.com
17. www.foodproductiondaily.com/news 20/09/2005
18. www.foodproductiondaily.com/news 08/02/2006
19. Sick Of Pesticides Campaign:
www.wen.org.uk/general_pages/Newsitems/pr_sickofpesticides23.3.09.doc
20. International Journal Occupational Environmental Health, Vol. 10, pages 468- 470, 2004.
21. http://www.choice.com.au/articles/a101575p12.htm
22. www.pan-uk.org/index.html
23. www.epa.gov/pesticides/factsheets/ipm.htm
24. www.pan-uk.org/projects/food/index.htm

25. Kroll and colleagues. Reduction of pesticide residues on produce by rinsing. Journal of Agriculture and Food Chemistry, Vol. 48, pages 4666-4670, 2000.
26. www.epa.gov/opp00001 /food/tips.html
27. www.articlebase.com/decontamination-of-pesticide-residues-on-fruit-and-vegetables-317329.html
28. J. Agriculture Food Chemistry, Vol. 50, pages 3412-3418, 2002.

Chapter 5

29. www.food.gov.uk/safereating/chemsafe/additivesbranch/enumberlist
30. Mozaffarian, and colleagues. Trans fatty acids and cardiovascular disease. New England Journal of Medicine, Vol. 354, pages 1601–1613, 2006.
31. McCann and colleagues, The Lancet, Vol. 370, pages 1560 - 1567, 2007.
32. www.moniqa.org/pre/13-Uygun-Food
33. The Food Magazine, March 10th 2007, reported free at news.scotsman.com/gmfood/Alarm-over-banned-food-additives.3353241.jp
34. Ferrand and colleagues, Journal Agriculture Food Chemistry, Vol. 48, pages 3605–3610, 2000.
35. Piper, Free Radical Biology Medicine, Vol. 27 pages 1219–27, 1999.
36. Arranz and colleagues, Toxicology in Vitro, Vol. 21, pages 1311-1317, 2007.
37. Mukherjee and Chakrabarti, Food and Chemical Toxicology, Vol. 35, pages 1177-1179, 1997.
38. Soffritti and colleagues, Environmental Health Perspectives, Vol. 115, pages 1293–1297, 2007.
39. Collison and colleagues, Journal Lipid Research, (www.jlr.org/cgi/reprint/M800418-LR200v1.pdf)
40. Hermanussen and Tresguerres, European Journal Clinical Nutrition, Vol.60, pages 25-31, 2006.

Chapter 6

41. www.wwf.org.uk/filelibrary/pdf/biomonitoringresults.pdf
42. www.ewg.org/reports
43. Soni and colleagues, Food and Chemical Toxicology, Vol.43, pages 985-1015, 2005.
44. www.cosmeticsdatabase.co
45. Fruijtier-Polloth, Toxicology, Vol. 214, pp. 1-38, 2005, access at: Linkinghub.elsevier.com/retrieve/pii/S0300483X05002696
46. Bertazzi and colleagues, American Journal of Epidemiology Vol. 153, pages 1031-1044, 2001.
47. www.statcan.gc.ca/survey/household/measures/measures-mesures-eng.htm
48. www.biomonitoringinfo.org/new/20051128.html
49. www.wwf.org.uk/filelibrary/pdf/biomonitoringresults.pdf
50. www.ewg.org/sites/humantoxome/
51. http://cot.food.gov.uk/cotreports/cotwgreports/cocktailreport
52. http://cot.food.gov.uk/cotreports/cotcomcocannreps/cotcomcocrep2004
53. www.americanchemistry.com/s_acc/sec_acc_rcol.asp
54. http://assets.panda.org/downloads/12_pager_summary.pdf
55. Lau and colleagues, Toxicological Sciences, Vol. 90, pages 178-187, 2006.
56. www.food.gov.uk/news/newsarchive/2006/benzenesurvey
57. Laetz and colleagues, Environ. Health Perspect. Vol. 117, pages 348-353, 2009.
58. info.cancerresearchuk.org/cancerstats/types/testis/incidence
59. Sheikh and colleagues, J. Royal Society Medicine, Vol. 101, pages 139-143, 2008.
60. European Environment Agency Report No.10/2005, www.eea.europa.eu/publications/eea_report_2005_10

61. www.wen.org.uk with ref. 62 for names of suppliers of toxin-free cosmetics
62. www.devdelay.org/newsletter/articles/html/323-personal-care-products
63. www.ewg.org/Healthy-Home-Tips-01 for safety review of cosmetics
64. www.ewg.org/reports/teens
65. www.epa.gov/kidshometour
66. www.greenshop.co.uk
67. www.who.int/mediacentre/factsheets/fs225/en/index.html
68. Josef Krop, Healing the Planet, One Patient at a Time. A Primer in Environmental Medicine, 1997, (ISBN 0-9731945-0-2).
69. Schecter, Chemosphere, vol. 37, issue 9-12, pages 1807-1816, October 1998.
70. Dahlgren, Chemosphere, Volume 69, Issue 8, October 2007, Pages 1320-1325.
71. Wisner and colleagues, Treatment of children with detoxification method developed by Hubbard, Proc. Amer. Public Health Assoc. National Conference, 1995.
72. Rapp, D.J. "Our Toxic World A Wakeup Call", 2004, see: www.drrapp.com/publications.htm
73. "Child-specific Exposure Factors Handbook", 2008, U.S.A. Environmental Protection Agency, Washington, USA.
74. "What's Really in Your Basket? An Easy Guide to Food additives and Cosmetics Ingredients, by Bill Statham, Summersdale Pub. 2007.
75. Richardson, A. "They Are What You Feed Them", 2006, see: www.fabresearch.org/view_item.aspx?item_id=960

Chapter 7

76. www.prnewswire.co.uk/cgi/news/release?id=96968
77. British Association of Parental and Enteral Nutrition (BAPEN) report, 2005, www.bapen.org.uk
78. Joanne Blythman, "The Food We Eat" (Michael Joseph 1996).
79. Joanne Blythman, "Bad Food Britain: How A Nation Ruined Its Appetite" (Fourth Estate 2006).
80. www.food.gov.uk/foodindustry/famingfood/organicfood
81. Organic Food: Facts and Figures, 2006, www.soilassociation.org
82. www.food.gov.uk/news/newsarchive/2009
83. Dangour and colleagues, American Journal Clinical Nutrition, Vol. 90, pages 680-685, 2009.
84. Mozaffarian and colleagues, Journal American Medical Assoc., Vol. 289, pages 1659-1666, 2003.
85. "Irradiated Food in Europe and the UK", The Food Commission, July 2002, www.foodcomm.org.uk/irradiation_probs.htm
86. Giannakourou and Taoukis, Food Chemistry, Vol. 83, pages 33-41, 2003.
87. Vallejo and colleagues, Journal of the Science of Food and Agriculture, Vol. 83, pages 1511-1516, 2003.
88. http://ods.od.nih.gov
89. lpi.oregonstate.edu/infocenter
90. www.food.gov.uk/multimedia/webpage/vitandmin/ Then open up pdf entitled "Safe upper limits for vitamins and minerals, 2003".
91. Jenkins and colleagues, Canadian Medical Association Journal fact sheet, 2008, see: www.cmaj.ca/cgi/content/full/178/2/150

Chapter 8

92. www.netdoctor.co.uk/dietandnutriton/feature/vitamins
93. www.food.gov.uk/science/dietarysurveys/ndnsdocuments
94. www.5aday.nhs.uk Open up "The school fruit and vegetable scheme".
95. Hypponen and Power, Journal Clinical Nutrition, Vol. 85, pages 860-868, 2007.

96. Lavie and colleagues, Journal American College of Cardiology, Vol. 54, pages 585-594, 2009.
97. www.food.gov.uk/science/surveillance/fsis2003/fsis402003
98. Ann Intern Med. 2006;145:364-371.
99. www.ajcn.org/cgi/reprint/85/1/265S.pdf?ck=nck
100. Stidley, Cancer Research, Vol.70, pages 568-574, 2010.
101. http://www.food.gov.uk/multimedia/pdfs/vitmin2003.pdf
102. Pauling L. "How to Live Longer and Feel Better", New York: WH Freeman, 1986.

103. Orr and Sohal, Science, Vol. 263, pages 1128-1130, 1994.
104. news.bbc.co.uk/2/hi/health/4520727

105. http://www.thecochranelibrary.com, 2009, issue 1, Nikolova and colleagues.
106. Tucker, American Journal Clinical Nutrition, Vol. 71, pages 514-522, 2000.
107. Wald and colleagues, British Medical Journal, Vol. 333, pages 1114-1117.
108. Tat and colleagues, Arthritis Research Therapy, 9, R117, 2007.
109. Bijlsma and Lafeber, Annals Internal Medicine, Vol. 148, pages 315-316, 2008.
110. www.nutrition.org.uk/home

111. Reaves and colleagues, J. American Dietetic Association, Vol. 106, pages 2018-2023, 2006.
112. Das and colleagues, Archives Disease in Childhood, Vol. 91, pages 569-572, 2006.
113 Vieth, editorial in American Journal of Clinical Nutrition, Vol. 85, pages 649-650, 2007.
114. Gariballa, British Medical Journal, Vol. 331, pages 304-305, 2005.
115. Lesourd, American Journal Clinical Nutrition, Vol. 66, pages 478s-484s, 1997.
116. Durga and colleagues, Lancet, Vol. 369, pages 208-216, 2007. If you do not subscribe to Lancet, scan down the top page of search engine and you will find the article extracted by other links.
117. Autier, Archives of Internal Medicine, Vol. 167, 1730-1737, 2007 see, archinte.ama-assn.org/content/vol167/issue16/index.dtl
118. Whalley, American Journal of Clinical Nutrition, Vol. 87, pages 449-454, 2008.
119. Hsia, Calcium/vitamin D supplementation and cardiovascular events, Circulation, Vol. 115, pages 846-854, 2007.
120. Bruno, Free Radical Biology and Medicine, Vol. 40, pages 689-697, 2006.
121. Duara and colleagues, presentation at American Academy Neurology, 60th Anniversary Annual Meeting, Chicago, USA, April 16th, 2008.
122. www.medscape.com/viewarticle/573383
123. Thornalley and colleagues, Diabetologia, Vol. 50, pages 2164-2170, 2007.
124. Head and Jurenka, Alternative Medicine Review, Vol. 9, pages 360-401, 2004.
125. Hypponen and Power, Diabetes Care, Vol. 29, pages 2244-2246, 2006.
126. www.pponline.co.uk/encyc/supplements-athletes.html

127. www.food.gov.uk, and open up "July 2008 EC update on vitamins and minerals in food".

Additional Useful References on Vitamins

128. The British Menopause Society: Fact Sheets. British Menopause Society 4-6 Eton Place, Marlow, Buckinghamshire, UK, SL7 2QA. Tel. +44 (0) 1628 890199, Fax: +44 (0) 1628 474042.
129. Wang, and colleagues, present evidence of the benefits of fish oil in cardiovascular disease. American Journal of Clinical Nutrition, Vol. 84, pages 5-17, 2006.
130. Lavie and colleagues, present mounting evidence for fish oils not only preventing heart disease but also reducing mortalities in patients with heart disease. Journal of American College of Cardiology, Vol. 54, pages 585-594, 2009.
131. Dijkstra and colleagues, cast some doubt on benefits of fish oils. European Journal of Heart Failure, Vol. 11, pages 922-928, 2009.
132. The American Journal of Clinical Nutrition –very useful specialist information on latest research on Vitamins: www.ajcn.org
133. www.medicinenet.com is very useful for information on vitamins.

Chapter 9

134. Church and Blair, British Journal of Sports Medicine, Vol. 43, pages 80-81, 2009.
135. Kujala, British Journal of Sports Medicine, Vol. 43, pages 550-555, 2009.
136. Hakim and colleagues. Effects of walking on mortality among non-smoking retired men, New England Journal of Medicine, Vol. 338, pages 94-99, 1998.

Chapter 11

137. **www.csp.org.uk/uploads/documents/csp_lazy_exercise_leaflet.pdf**
138. **www.netdoctor.co.uk/pelvicexercise**
139. **www.ic.nhs.uk/ncmp**
140. Schrager, Journal Applied Physiology, Vol. 102, pages 919-925, 2007.
141. **www.nia.nih.gov/exercise** (click on Chapter 4, "Sample Exercises-Strength")